PRAI

In Due Time: A Jou

Loss, and Embracing the Unknown

"I am so thankful for the bravery and candor that Jen puts into every single word of *In Due Time*. In an age when people seem to be able to have everything that they desire, infertility is still a painful, often secret reality for many couples who desperately wait for children. Whether you are struggling through infertility, or your infertility journey is complete, you will find a kindred spirit in these pages."

- Matt Appling, co-author of
*Plus or Minus: Keeping Your Life, Faith
and Love Together Through Infertility*

"Jen writes with courage and honesty that will resonate with many women struggling to achieve their dream of a child. *In Due Time* provides helpful coping skills that can be useful for anyone facing life challenges. The author's journey is told in a very easy to read manner that will make you laugh and make you cry and in the end make you rejoice with her."

- Judy Becerra, LPC,
Colorado Center for Reproductive Medicine

"Jen shares her journey through infertility and loss with vulnerability and honesty. Whether you are newly diagnosed or an IVF vet, you will find more similarities to your own story than differences."

- Jessica Martin,
blogger at *A Hummingbird Paused*

"*In Due Time* is equal parts information and inspiration! If you're walking your own journey towards motherhood through infertility Jen's experience will help you every step of the way. She uses humour and incredible candour while explaining every feeling, physical and emotional, she has experienced to get to her happy ending. Jen has a wonderful way of making you feel that you ARE normal with all of the crazy that can surround you during infertility and treatment and that is no small feat! I highly recommend this book along with a box of Kleenex, you will cry along with her through sadness as well as joy."

- Kaeleigh MacDonald,
blogger at *Unpregnant Chicken*

"*In Due Time* is a raw, straightforward memoir providing a greater understanding of the rollercoaster of infertility. Jen's words connect deeply with anyone who has struggled. Her memoir is relatable, educational and inspiring, and a must read for anyone struggling, supporting or wanting to learn more about infertility. Plan to settle in - you won't be able to put it down!"

- Chelsea Ritchie, blogger at
Starbucks, Peace, and the Pursuit of a Baby

In Due Time

In Due Time

A Journey Through Infertility, Loss, and Embracing the Unknown

JEN NOONAN

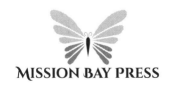

MISSION BAY PRESS

In Due Time: A Journey Through Infertility, Loss, and Embracing the Unknown
Published by Mission Bay Press
Denver, CO

Library of Congress Control Number: 2015938647
Noonan, Jen, Author
In Due Time: A Journey Through Infertility, Loss,
and Embracing the Unknown
Jen Noonan

ISBN: 978-0-9963086-0-1

HEALTH & FITNESS / Infertility

QUANTITY PURCHASES: Schools, companies, professional groups, clubs, and other organizations may qualify for special terms when ordering quantities of this title. For information, email info@MissionBayPress.com.

This book is printed in the United States of America.

To my husband, Patrick,
my rock through a rocky journey.

Author's Note

The events depicted in this book are authentic and the people are real. In most instances the names are real, but some have been changed out of respect for privacy. All conversations are real, and have been reconstructed to the best of my recollection.

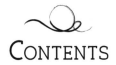

CONTENTS

PREFACE

This book emerged while I was struggling to accept one of many failed infertility treatments. I turned to my husband, Patrick and said, "I have to write a book about all we've experienced." I assumed writing a book would be therapeutic, and would inspire those who have experienced, are currently experiencing, or might experience something similar. I also realized how little many of my friends, family, and acquaintances knew about infertility, and I wished to shine a light on what many of us consider the most challenging time of our lives. I kept a daily journal of infertility treatments and the feelings associated with them, as I went along.

As I began to write the book, I took into consideration the plethora of infertility books, and wondered how I could make mine stand out from the others. Most infertility books focused specifically on the Western medical viewpoint, the emotional challenges (how to cope), or the nutritional / alternative strategies to successfully conceive.

Infertility memoirs seemed to be in short supply, specifically ones that gave an account of an entire journey of ups and downs, from start to finish. Although every person's journey is unique, similar themes seem to appear in each of our stories. I strived to share the unpleasant and chaotic lifestyle that those of us struggling with infertility experience, as well as a few moments of grace.

Because I am a Licensed Professional Counselor, I agonized over the thought of clients reading about the many times I became unhinged. At the other extreme, I worried that people still struggling with infertility would find fault with my triumphs. I finally decided to opt for vulnerability and transparency. I've done my best to share with you an honest account. My only hope is that I have created a source of hope that is credible, relatable, raw and honest.

1
NEW ZEALAND

"As long as your happiness is caused or sustained by something or someone outside of you, you are still in the land of the dead. The day you are happy for no reason whatsoever, the day you find yourself taking delight in everything and in nothing, you will know that you have found the land of unending joy called the kingdom."
                                                    - Fr. Anthony DeMello

D ad, I'm so confused!" I cried eight thousand miles away in New Zealand.

"What do you mean?" he asked.

"I thought traveling the world, living in another country, and discovering myself was a solid plan. I thought I was too young to get a real job and start a career after graduation. But now I'm twenty-four, and I feel like I've fallen behind."

"Think of the experiences you've gained by living in other countries, and how valuable that will be for your future," he replied.

"Yeah, but all my friends have started on their career path and gained professional experience. I'll have to start from the beginning, and I'm scared I've wasted too much time."

"I'm sure you'll be just fine," my dad said.

I hung up the phone feeling defeated and second-guessing the decisions I made.

I had embarked on an around-the-world journey almost two years prior, with the intention of living and working in New Zealand for one year. The year turned into nearly two as I sought permanent residency to stay longer. It was a place I envisioned growing old in. I adored this picturesque country and its amiable people, despite the frequent damp and dreary weather. However, I felt isolated and lonely. Both of my flat mates were New Zealand natives and had family and friends nearby. Although I had formed a small group of friends, I didn't feel as connected to the country as I hoped, and I began to consider packing up my belongings and moving home.

Before making a decision, I needed to think about my options. Everything I did up to that point had been planned out to avoid surprises. Although I liked adventure, I was not a risk-taker. I preferred to move only with a carefully laid out plan. My decision to move back to the States after almost two years of living in another country was no exception.

I strolled the short distance down the hill from our house to Mission Bay, where I often went to contemplate important decisions. I sat at the water's edge, pulled out my journal, and began listing pros and cons for returning home or remaining in New Zealand. I recalled all the adventures I had experienced since arriving. I had bungee-jumped, skydived, and paraglided. I had walked the land where The *Lord of the Rings* was filmed. I had visited deserted beaches. I had engaged in colorful conversations and established friendships with people from all corners of the world. However, I felt too distanced from friends and family. New Zealand was a sixteen-hour plane ride from my home state of Illinois. I pondered where I might live, and what kind of job I would seek if I did return home. After the list of pros for returning home became longer than the list for staying, I packed up my journal and walked back to my house with a heavy heart.

One month before I left New Zealand, I was introduced to Susanna, a fellow traveler who had been living and working in the South Island. She was on her way back home to Denver via Auckland, and needed a place to stay for the night. We had an extensive conversation on my front porch regarding where I would live when I returned home.

"I just can't imagine living in Chicago again," I said. "The bars and restaurants are exiting, and the summer activities along the lakeshore are unbeatable, but I can't tolerate the flat streets, lack of nature, bitterly cold winters, and gray skies."

"I grew up in New Mexico, but when my brother moved to Denver, I started thinking about moving there as well. It's nice to have family nearby."

"I've never been to Colorado. What's Denver like?" I asked.

"You would love it! The Rocky Mountains are spectacular, and there are so many places to go hiking. It's one of the sunniest cities in the States, and I hear there are four guys to every one girl, so the dating scene is ideal!" she said. "I have an extra bedroom in my house that you're welcome to rent while you look for a permanent place. I have someone living in the basement of the house, and we have two dogs. Hopefully, that's not a problem."

"A problem? I love dogs! I've just always felt too free-spirited to get one. I don't know anyone in Denver, so the more roommates, the better. I guess the downside to moving away from Chicago would be leaving friends and family. I'll have to think about all of this and let you know," I said.

I felt energized by my conversation with Susanna, and spent a few days researching Denver, imagining what it might feel like to live there. I hunted for jobs, researched moving costs, and found things to do and see in the surrounding area. As exciting as it seemed, I still wasn't ready to commit, so I began to prepare to move back to Chicago.

I sold most of the belongings I had accumulated over the years: a car, bed, dresser, desk, bed linens, and cell phone. As ready as I was to move forward in life, I didn't anticipate the sadness I would feel about letting go of my few possessions and saying goodbye to friends and acquaintances. My co-workers threw a goodbye party for me and wished me the best.

On the Air New Zealand flight bound for Tahiti, I was unable to stop crying. A baby screamed, the cabin sweltered, and I became increasingly irritated. I berated myself for not being courageous enough to overcome the loneliness and isolation of living in New Zealand. I was disappointed with myself for having pursued a residency permit that would be wasted. I became discouraged at the thought of returning home with two suitcases, no job, no boyfriend, and no permanent place to live. I had been meticulous about executing my plans in the past. This one hadn't worked, and I was not pleased.

2
FINDING "THE ONE"

"When you've integrated the bliss, happiness, and goodness of your soul, you can easily manifest the wonderful results you want in your life because your thoughts, beliefs, and feelings have come into alignment and harmony with your true goals."

- Jonathan Parker

When I returned to Chicago, I half-heartedly sought to find a job and settle down, believing it was easier than moving. But after a few months of doing temporary work, I became disenchanted. I reached out to Susanna and moved to Denver.

Two days after my arrival, Susanna introduced me to a group of her friends at a pub in Denver. Her girlfriends were warm and welcoming. Her guy friends were lively and entertaining. One guy friend in particular, Patrick, captured my attention with his genuine smile and soft blue eyes. He had a quirky sense of humor, and I discovered we had a lot of common interests. He appeared to be down to earth, smiled a lot, and was easy to talk with. He invited some of the group back to his house.

Patrick lived in a neighborhood called Washington Park that I was not familiar with, having been in Denver for a short time. Susanna explained it was a highly desirable place to live.

"When did you move here?" I asked Patrick.

"I bought the house in 1998, but it looked nothing like it does today. The kitchen was pink, and there was shag carpeting in the basement bedroom! There was even a dishwasher on wheels that I had to roll over to the sink to use! I finished remodeling it just before you moved here."

As I looked around the tastefully decorated house, I couldn't imagine its prior look.

"What prompted you to remodel it?" I asked.

"Well, that's a bit of a long story," he said.

"Try me," I encouraged.

"I was engaged to someone, but it fell apart about a year ago. I guess we just wanted different things. It forced me to do things I might not have done had I stayed with her, such as this remodel. I wanted to set up my house to allow the right person to come into my life and settle here with me."

"Sometimes things happen for the best," I said.

The more we talked, the more I learned.

Patrick grew up in Southern California, approximately twenty minutes inland from Malibu, where his parents still lived. He didn't strike me as someone who came from that part of the country. He didn't look like any of the characters on Beverly Hills 90210 that I crushed on back in the day.

He was tall and slender with brown hair and striking blue eyes, but he didn't appear preoccupied with material things or his appearance. He had a younger brother living in Santa Monica, and a younger sister living in Lake Tahoe.

Patrick took me on my first snowboarding adventure to Copper Mountain. He patiently waited while I flipped and fell across the mountain. He had learned to ski as a child on family vacations to Park City, Utah, and he could breeze down advanced runs. That day he supported me by providing pointers regarding dismounting the chair lift successfully. As my snowboard dangled from my right foot, I tried desperately to place my left foot on the board, stand up, and slide forward without plowing into anyone. It was a wobbly attempt, but I managed to not embarrass myself.

The drive from Copper Mountain back to Denver allowed me to get to know Patrick even better.

"What brought you out here?" I asked.

"An enticing job opportunity that I couldn't pass up. That's where I met Susanna," he said. "We worked at a company called Convergent Group where I was a geographic information systems consultant. I recently started my own business, though. It was something I had been thinking about for a while. I think the breakup with my fiancé propelled me forward with my goals."

Over the years, Patrick and I became closer. Our shared love of travel took us to Mexico, Canada, and Costa Rica. Our shared love of music took us to many concerts at local venues. Although there was an obvious physical and emotional attraction, we never formed an official romantic relationship. This changed when I contacted him after breaking off a year-long relationship. We had not spoken in more than a year when I found the courage to email him.

"Hey, Stranger. It's been a while, hasn't it? I was thinking what good friends we once were, and how this lack of communication has been somewhat silly. How would you feel about getting together for lunch one of these days to catch up?"

My hands shook as his reply came through the same day.

"Wow, great to hear from you. I agree, it's been too long and I have actually entertained thoughts of getting back in touch with you lately. (Funny how you thought the same.) I would be up for lunch or dinner. I don't have firm plans for this weekend. What do you think?"

We met up for dinner, and there was no denying the physical and emotional connection anymore. I had missed him tremendously.

"So what's changed since we last hung out?" he asked.

"Well, I am about halfway through a master's degree in counseling psychology at the University of Colorado Denver," I explained.

"That's great," he said. "You had always talked about your goal of getting a master's degree!"

"Yes. That was on my list. I've always been a planner," I said. "I make goals for one year, five years, and ten years out, and do my best to accomplish them."

"Have you mostly been successful?" he asked.

"For the most part, yes, I have," I said, although at the moment, I felt I was far off from operating at my peak. I wasn't sure where the degree would lead me, and knew it would not be useful for advancement at my current job where

I sent college students to study abroad in Australia and New Zealand.

"So what's left on your list of goals?" Patrick asked.

"That's simple. I want to start a career using my counseling degree, get married, live in a family-friendly neighborhood, spend time with friends and family, and have two children, preferably a boy and a girl. Do you think that's too much to ask?" I joked.

"It all seems attainable to me," he responded, "but I thought you said you weren't sure you wanted kids."

"You're right. I did say that. I don't have a younger sibling, and most of my cousins are my age or older, so I never grew up around a baby or young kids. I also don't feel that my mom taught me how to be a good parent, and I was always concerned that I might not be a good one."

"But you feel differently now?"

"If I married the right person, and could provide a baby with a financially stable, loving home, yes, I would want to have children," I said. "I've often thought about how exciting it would be to re-experience childhood adventures with your own kids, and how fun it would be to see how much they look like you."

"That's good to know," Patrick said. "I've always wanted kids...with the right person."

3

FALLING INTO PLACE

*"Happiness often sneaks in through a door
you didn't know you left open."*

- John Barrymore

Patrick asked me to fly to California to meet his parents for Thanksgiving 2007. I wondered what they would be like and hoped they would like me. Patrick warned me that his dad might grill me about my education and career, because these things were of interest to him. He countered with a description of his mom as someone who has a great sense of humor, who would put me at ease. I was nervous, but looked forward to this milestone in our relationship.

Patrick's mom, Sandy, picked us up at the airport with a welcoming grin and a friendly hug. "Welcome to California Jen!" She took us back to the house the family had moved to when Patrick was ten. Patrick's dad, Pat, greeted me with a warm hug as well, and eventually began questioning me. "Where did you go to undergrad?" he asked.

"The University of Illinois in Champaign-Urbana. I hear you went to the University of Michigan. Go Big Ten!" I hoped I had scored a point with him!

He laughed and shouted "Go Blue!" He then asked "What are you doing for work at the moment?"

"I work at a company called AustraLearn, where I send students to study abroad in New Zealand and Australia."

"Patrick mentioned you lived in New Zealand. That must be a rewarding job."

"It is, but I'm also in the process of getting a master's degree in counseling psychology," I said.

"How did you make that decision?" he asked.

"I've always been interested in psychology, but never pursued it. I'm fascinated with the challenges people face in life, and enjoy helping friends with their struggles. I think what really drove me into the field, unfortunately, was the strained relationship I have with my mom. I want to learn why people think the way they do, and do the things they do."

"Sorry to hear about the relationship. I wish you the best with finishing the degree," Pat said.

The rest of the visit was filled with Sandy's delectable cooking, stimulating conversation, and excellent wine. Sandy and Pat were gracious hosts, and I looked forward to getting to know them more.

On April 20, 2008, Patrick and I took a walk in Washington Park, one of our favorite places to relax. He suggested we walk to the end of the dock overlooking the lake on the south side of the park. When we got close to the spot, he said "We've known each other for a long time…" and that's all I remember. My gut told me what was about to happen, and I felt like I couldn't breathe. I was overwhelmed with joy, for this was the man I had wanted to be with for the rest of my life since I had first gotten to know him five years earlier. He led me to the end of the dock, got down on one knee, and asked me to marry him. It seemed life was unfolding with ease.

My soon to be mother-in-law, Sandy, offered to help with the preparations in any way possible, so I asked her for help with the rehearsal dinner. She and Pat flew in for a visit, and we toured multiple venues before settling on the perfect one.

"I really appreciate your stepping in to help us, Sandy."

"Jen, you don't know how long we've waited for Patrick to get married," she joked. "We're so happy for the two of you, and we're thrilled you'll be joining our family."

The wedding day soon approached, and we celebrated with our very closest friends and family at various locations around the city. I did my best to ignore the fact that my mother didn't participate in any of the pre-wedding events such as the engagement party, dress shopping, venue and food decisions, and wedding shower. Our relationship had been strained for such a long time that it seemed natural that I would make these decisions with my fiancé and our friends.

However, the more I tried to suppress my sorrow and anger, the more I felt it.

Our wedding day was a beautiful October celebration. We got married at a church across the street from Washington Park (where we had gotten engaged), and had the reception at a historic mansion in a nearby neighborhood. I heeded the advice of many by taking a moment to relish the scene of everyone gathered to celebrate our marriage. I couldn't stop smiling. Although the front page of the Denver Post read "Worst Week Ever" due to the 2008 financial crisis, I felt like my life was coming together even better than I had anticipated.

We spent an adventure-filled week honeymooning in Tahiti where we snorkeled, rode ATVs, relaxed on the balcony of our over-the-water bungalow, and kayaked. While viewing the breathtaking sunset one night, I said to my new husband, "I think I've done it all."

When we returned to Colorado, Patrick was informed that his consulting contract hours for the City and County of Charlotte, North Carolina, would significantly decrease. The 2008 financial crisis (considered the worst since the Great Depression) had affected many jobs, and his was not spared. He had purchased a distressed house in a neighboring city a few years prior that he had been renting. He soon became aware of the large number of foreclosed and short sale properties, and he decided to take advantage of the situation by buying and holding. My full-time job and the income from the rental properties would keep us afloat.

About three months into our marriage, I brought up the topic of having children. I surprised myself with how soon I decided it was time to start a family.

"I know we've been married for a short time, but I'm thirty-two and you're forty," I said. "We're both obviously healthy, so there shouldn't be a problem, but we have to consider how old we'll be when trying for a second. I am well aware that plenty of thirty-five-plus-year-olds don't have children with genetic abnormalities, but the chances do increase the older you are."

"I'm thinking more about how long it would be before we could retire and travel!" Patrick joked.

"Yeah, there's also that to think about, and also how old *you* would be when they graduate high school. You'd be close to sixty-two when the second one graduates!" I laughed.

I put on my visioning hat, and began to create a plan to get pregnant, complete my hours to become a licensed professional counselor, quit my job, and become a stay-at-home mom. I had never imagined being a stay-at-home mom, but knew it would be more enjoyable than the daily frustration and exhaustion of my job. I had been working at a nonprofit agency as a case manager for nurses with substance abuse and dependence diagnoses. Although I was using my counseling degree, the job responsibilities took an emotional and physical toll on my well-being.

I visited a primary care physician for my annual exam, and announced that I wanted to stop taking birth control pills. She encouraged me to wait at least a month after stopping birth control to try to get pregnant, as many women conceive during this time, and birth defects sometimes occur due to residual effects. I didn't see any reason to wait. I assumed those kinds of things happen to other people, not me. I was healthy, and I had no concerns about whether or not I would get pregnant or how it would go. I was a prime candidate to become pregnant easily. I was 5 feet 1 inch tall and 114 pounds, I ate mostly healthy foods, drank alcohol moderately, didn't take prescription medication, took my daily supplements, and was never diagnosed with a major illness. The only surgery I'd had was wisdom teeth removal. My period arrived every single month like clockwork since it had started. My blood pressure was normal, and my mother conceived two children just over three years apart without any challenges.

4
FAMILY PLANNING

"Nature knows all about timing and exists accordingly, in a state of balance and vitality. As forces of nature ourselves, we must learn to do the same. No matter how much we desire a certain life, a particular role, a specific reward for efforts made, if the conditions are not in place for those results to arise we will not get what we desire. Not because we don't deserve it, but because our desire is less important than the balance of the cosmos and the integrity of the living, breathing organism that is this planet."

- Sarah Varcas

MONTH 1

The first week in February 2009, we began trying to conceive. I documented it in my journal:

February 5, 2009

Today I feel more alive than I have in a while. Maybe it was the doctor visit yesterday to discuss planning a family. Maybe I need to move on to the next chapter in my life. Maybe it feels good to have something positive to think about when work is challenging. Maybe it was the dinner we had out last night and I feel like we're "living" again despite the economic downturn.

It didn't seem odd to me that we did not conceive that month, but it did seem odd that my cycle was shorter than usual, only twenty-four days in length. I attributed this to having gone off birth control, and my body being slightly out of whack. I was disappointed, but looked forward to giving it another try in March.

We went to Mexico with my in-laws, Sandy and Pat. We hadn't told them we were trying to have a baby, and didn't plan to. I considered myself somewhat of an open book, but didn't feel like discussing anything pregnancy-related until it actually happened. We spent an adventure-filled week a short distance from Playa del Carmen. We toured the ancient ruins of Tulum and lounged around the pool at a water park / zoo called Xcaret. It was exhilarating to be traveling again, experiencing a different culture.

MONTH 2

March 30, 2009

"Slightly disappointed to have gotten my period today, but I can't stress over it. I'm doing everything the web sites say to do."

When I got my period again, I was disappointed and went on a fact-finding mission with Google. *What was it that Google said about how many months it should take to conceive if you're younger than thirty-five years old?* I ran to my computer to check. The only information I could find said, "If you're under thirty-five and you haven't conceived after a year, you should see your primary care physician or a reproductive endocrinologist (RE)."

I became concerned as I continued reading. I discovered that after age thirty, the chances of conceiving in any given month diminish, and they fall further as you get older, dropping steeply in your forties. I figured I had about a 10 to 15 percent chance of conceiving during any given cycle, which seemed to be low odds. But we had just started trying, and it had not yet been a year. I assured myself it would happen in the next few months.

I had been taking a class called "Beyond Limits" at Mile Hi Church, a spiritual center just outside of Denver with a Science of Mind philosophy. We were asked to write our intentions for the ten-week class. I wrote, "My intention for this class is being able to focus on growth and development in the areas of confidence and self-esteem. My intention is to become more self-assured in the decisions I make, and to learn new ways of thinking to result in improved relationships with friends, family, and co-workers. Most importantly, my intention is to develop tools and skills to be a nurturing and caring future mother."

In an exercise titled, "Six Questions to Focus Your Life," I was asked what great thing I would give to my life if I were absolutely assured of success. I answered, "A child – I am concerned about my ability to parent."

In the exercise, "Something I Want for My Life," I answered, "I desire a healthy child within the next year." When asked how I block this desire, I answered, "I block this by being overly concerned if I will be able to conceive, when I'll be able to, and what kind of a mother I will be."

My mom and I had a difficult and volatile relationship throughout most of my childhood. She gave little encouragement or affection and tended to focus on criticizing me instead. She did not mentor me about puberty and boys, or about applying makeup. She did not support me at after-school events. I never felt like I was "enough." From the time I was eleven years old, I cycled through periods of anxiety and depression. I tried to understand the reasons behind my mother's behavior. She, too, had experienced a "cold and unloving" upbringing. I became concerned that I would follow the pattern of mothering that had existed in my family for generations.

My maternal grandparents lived approximately a thirty-minute drive from my childhood home. I do not remember my grandfather ever visiting our house, nor did we ever visit my grandparents at their house. I recall one unexpected visit when my grandmother drove to our house without my grandfather and brought me a Mickey Mouse toy. This is one of my only memories of ever seeing my grandmother. Despite receiving birthday cards from my grandparents with money tucked inside, I grew up without any contact from them. My parents never explained why my brother and I never saw our grandparents, so I was left to conclude that they did not want to spend time with us. My mom's sister and brother had moved out of state as young adults, and we did not have a relationship with them, which meant I did not know my cousins either. The women in my immediate and extended family on my mom's side were emotionally and physically unavailable. Upon closer examination, I believe I grew up with an underlying feeling of rejection, not knowing why.

Continuing on with the exercises in the course, the next field asked us to describe a hidden belief we have about health and body. I wrote, "The part of my body that is trying to give me a message is my uterus. It's telling me to relax. A baby will be created when it's the right time. The uterus is telling me that I'm doing everything I should be doing to make this happen. Being anxious about it not happening, and treating it as if it is a to-do item that needs to be crossed off the list, is not beneficial."

I was then asked to write an Empowerment Belief to contradict my hidden belief. I wrote, "You are meant to be a mother and are going to be one very soon. You have treated your body with kindness and respect over the years and will therefore be rewarded. The body is ready to create a child, but wants to do so in its own time. It's okay if this doesn't happen right away, because, as has always been the case, things happen the way they should, and WHEN they should. Things always turn out okay."

MONTH 3

Three months of trying, and again I got my period. One of my husband's many cousins and his wife got pregnant two months after their wedding the previous year, and were about to have their baby. This was the first baby born in my extended family since we had started trying to conceive. I was overjoyed for them; yet I wondered when it would be our turn.

May 10, 2009

> *...why is it not happening? Is it due to something I've done in the past? Do I not deserve it? Is there something wrong with me? The stress and anxiety that has come along with this whole thing is not healthy, and I'm wondering if it's time to stop worrying about it. I continuously wonder if I'm ovulating. I have a few glasses of wine and I wonder if that has had an effect. I'm going crazy, and it needs to stop.*

A close friend gave me a book called *Taking Charge of Your Fertility* by Toni Weschler. She had received the book from her friend, but neither she nor her friend had had any problems conceiving, so the book was handed down to me. I read it cover to cover, paying special attention to the chapters that involved "Finally Making Sense of Your Menstrual Cycle," "The Three Primary Fertility Signs," "Anovulation," and "Irregular Cycles." The one about "Choosing the Sex of Your Baby" was entertaining and a nice break from the serious side of fertility. Weschler's book explained how to chart your menstrual cycle by taking your temperature daily, observing cervical mucus, and determining cervical position. I looked at all the examples of charts, and it seemed this activity would be too stressful for me. Besides, I was certain it was going to happen for us any month now, and charting would be a waste of time and energy.

Instead, I took a few notes for each day of my cycle, hoping to gather some insightful data, when I noticed a red flag. Throughout cycle days one to twenty, I mentioned, "light or very light sweating." It was not quite summer yet, so I didn't attribute this to the hot weather or my bedding. Google research indicated I might be experiencing perimenopause, and the worst-case scenario was that I had cancer, specifically leukemia. *Was it possible I was entering perimenopause at the ripe old age of thirty-two?* More than likely not, but it was something that needed to be considered.

May 12, 2009

Wow. How differently I'm looking at children now. I just have this yearning that I've never experienced before...I realize how stressed I've become over this. How much more relaxed I would feel if I knew this was taken care of. It's this ongoing anxiety about something I can't entirely control. And it's uncomfortable.

I signed up for a four-week Mindfulness Meditation course at the Colorado Free University. The class offered many tips on different styles of meditation and breathing, and I really latched on to the deep breathing method. Throughout the class, I tried to deep breathe and ignore any thoughts that popped into my head. The only downside to the class was that it was offered in the evenings after a long workday, and I found it challenging to stay awake.

Meanwhile, if I mentioned we were trying to get pregnant, people often would say, "Just relax, and it will happen." I dismissed my stress level as a cause. I knew it couldn't be attributed to that. After all, I was happily married and working at a job that paid me a decent salary. We had a lot of friends, we traveled, and we lived in a comfortable home. I *was* relaxed…other than feeling anxious that we had not yet conceived!

To help keep anxiety from moving in, I booked an appointment for a yearly physical with blood work to determine any possible contributing thyroid or hormonal issues. I also began using ovulation predictor kits (OPKs). These kits detect a rise in luteinizing hormone (LH), which happens twenty-four to thirty-six hours prior to ovulation. Unfortunately, I did not get a positive indicator that I was about to ovulate.

A few weeks passed, when I thought of a new idea. I would write in a journal to my unborn son or daughter. I believe a soul chooses its parents, and I wanted my future baby to know how much he or she was wanted. It felt a bit strange, but I began talking to the baby I hoped to meet some day.

MONTH 4

May 23, 2009

Dear Baby,

I made the decision to start this journal so we could begin this adventure together. The "Travel Diary" (on the front cover) fits perfectly, as this really IS a journey! I want to share all of my thoughts and experiences with you along the way. I'm hoping this will give me comfort and peace, and will one day be exciting for you to read!

I'll be the first to admit that I was never the person who was eager to have a child. In fact, I wasn't sure that I ever wanted one! I think a lot of that came from not having met the right person, but also I was afraid that I would end up treating a child like my mother had treated me. When your dad and I started dating, I knew the decision to have children was the right one, and I felt really good about it.

Today I found out that I am not pregnant with you yet. But I'm ready now. I am able to offer you a peaceful, relaxing, loving home. I am ready to love and cherish every day that you spend inside of me. We are able to offer you protection, kindness, love, and generosity. I am ready to be your mother, and your father is ready to be your father. I now understand that it's YOU who makes the choice when to come

into this world, not me. I will be here patiently waiting
for you to arrive.
With love,
Mom

So much for the meditation practice and the "patiently waiting" part that I had so lovingly written about in the baby journal. I could not accept that we had not become pregnant after four months. I went back to my primary care physician armed with questions. Why was I thirty-two years old, completely healthy, but not getting pregnant? I wanted an answer. I needed an answer, even if it hadn't been a year yet.

The day of my appointment fell on the twelfth day of my menstrual cycle. I later found out that most fertility testing is done on day three to achieve the most accurate results, but the general practitioner did not advise waiting until my next cycle. She referred me to a reproductive medicine facility called Colorado Center for Reproductive Medicine (CCRM), and specifically, Dr. William Schoolcraft. She explained that he was highly regarded in the field, and the facility had a high success rate. Although I was disappointed at not having conceived yet, I did not believe I was infertile, and I filed the referral away.

The practitioner did some blood work to test my hormone levels in a few areas key to fertility and mailed me a copy of my results with a message stating:

"Dear Jennifer, Your labs are normal. You are not in menopause. Your blood type is A-positive."

I did a double take and had to call the office to be sure they knew that I was, in fact, A-negative and not A-positive. I would later learn just how important that distinction is.

May 23, 2009

Finding out again that I'm not pregnant... I guess it's a feeling of "less than"...I KNOW in my heart there's a plan, a way that things are supposed to work. Timing will be the way it should be, and I'll look back and realize that it happened the way it should.

MONTH 5

I was headed toward a meltdown and couldn't convince myself to be patient. I couldn't focus on work and on nurturing friendships. Multiple times a day, I considered why this was happening. Was it some sort of karma? Did someone or something think I would not make a good parent?

I decided to have some fun and take a long travel break. Traveling always worked as a distraction. Due to 2009 being one of the worst economic years on record, flights to the South Pacific were cheap. Granted, it was off-season, but I was well aware of the beauty of the South Island of New Zealand during the winter, and I knew we would experience breathtaking views of mountains, fiords, lakes, and glaciers. Yes, it was time to get away, relax, have fun, and forget about the challenges of getting pregnant. There was always the chance it would happen while on holiday; what a story we would be able to tell! We booked our tickets to leave at the end of August, and counted the days until departure.

Meanwhile, I consulted with an herbalist for approximately ten sessions during which she addressed supplements and how to eat more wholesome foods. I increased my protein intake, and decreased my carbohydrate intake.

June 12, 2009

Dear Baby,

I spent time with Carrie last night, who is pregnant, asking her a lot of questions. She told me how she was able to feel her baby implanting into her uterus, and explained how. Now, I might just be imagining things, but I think I felt something similar today. I also (for the first time) had a dream that I was pregnant! And one more thing. Our cat jumped up on the couch as I was lying down, and decided to lie right on top of where I thought I felt you! But I've learned not to get too excited about these things, as I don't like to be disappointed. I can now only hope it's true. Awhile back, I bought a few books called "What to Expect When You're Expecting," and "The Pregnant Woman's Comfort Book." I hope to begin reading them really soon!

Something I haven't written about yet is all of the people who will be so excited about your arrival. Of course, your mom and dad, but also your grandparents!

I can't explain how much love and joy is waiting here for you. I promise that you will experience an abundance of it, and that we will do our best to provide you with the care and support you deserve every day of your life.

Love,

Mom

June 21, 2009

Dear Baby,

It's Father's Day, and I was hoping so much that I would NOT get my period today and that I would be pregnant with you, but unfortunately, that didn't happen. I was really disappointed yet again. I feel like, this time around, something was different, and maybe my body was trying to provide a safe place, but just wasn't able to. I know I need to be patient and to just relax, but it's such a challenge. I feel like I'm ready for this. I've come to realize that I'm doing everything I know how to do for this to happen. And that has to just be good enough for now. As always, I will be here waiting.

Love,

Mom

MONTH 6

Before we left on our New Zealand adventure, my menstrual cycle was approaching thirty-six days, and I just knew this would be our month. My cycle had never lasted longer than thirty-three days, so I figured it must mean it had finally happened. Patrick's birthday was coming up, and if all went well, my period would be late by almost a week on the morning of his birthday. I decided to take a pregnancy test that morning without telling him.

I held the pregnancy test in my hand and hoped beyond hope that it would be positive. I set the test on the counter top, and walked away. I like surprises. I cried when I was a child because I accidentally found the Christmas presents my dad had tried to hide so well. I waited for the maximum test time (about three minutes) before returning to check on the result.

Negative. Negative? My emotions plummeted. *What is wrong with this picture? What is wrong with ME? How amazing would it have been to find out on my husband's birthday that he would be a father? How fantastic would it have been to celebrate the news at one of the best restaurants in Denver? How incredible would it have felt to finally have conceived?* We managed to enjoy ourselves at dinner that night, and I was able to drink some exquisite wine, but the disappointing outcome was never far from my thoughts. My period eventually arrived after a forty-six day cycle—the longest I had ever experienced.

MONTH 7

August 2, 2009

Where did my period go? Why is my cycle off? Why do three tests show I'm not pregnant, but my period is two weeks late? The pregnancy challenge has just been bumped up a level. My periods have been regular since they began twenty-two years ago. What is going on? I'm tired of being so concerned. It's energy-draining, and I'm missing out on enjoying life. I should be looking forward to this great New Zealand trip coming up.

Seven months without a positive pregnancy test. Each cycle started out disappointing, with the arrival of my period, but then hope would build. I would think this was the magical month. I would count ahead nine months, and inevitably the due date would be close to a meaningful time in our lives. I would assume it was a sign. It just HAD to be a sign.

Periodically, people would ask, "When are you going to have kids?" That was the path we would have liked to take. However, this question never helped me feel better about our situation, and always reminded me what we didn't have. I would respond, "We'd like to. Someday."

August 16, 2009

Today marks the 1st day of the New Zealand trip. Sitting on this plane today, I can't help but think that when I was living in my "2nd home" (New Zealand), I had NO idea I'd be traveling back there with my husband. There were many things I didn't know would happen – loving Denver, running a marathon, grad school, buying a duplex, and of course the most incredible of all: meeting Patrick and eventually getting married. If there's anything all of this should have taught me, it's that you never know what's going to happen, that everything happens the way it should, and that amazing things are yet to come. I've decided to commit to a different and more positive attitude about the "unknown." It's going to be okay no matter what, just like it's always been. The more I attempt to control the future instead of letting things progress as they should, the

*more dis-ease I'm going to experience. When has my anxi-
ety been the lowest? When I live in the present moment
and let life flow.*

When we arrived in New Zealand, I took Patrick to my
past travel and living locations, and we relished the beauty
of the country. We walked by my old houses in the Mission
Bay and Ponsonby neighborhoods of Auckland, enjoyed dinner at the top of the Sky Tower with 360-degree views of
Auckland, spent a few days in Wellington, took a ferry to the
South Island, kayaked in Tasman Bay, jetboated in Queen-
stown, and rode bikes around the vineyards of the Marlbor-
ough wine region. I was relaxed and had so much fun that I
was certain it was going to happen for us.

When we returned to Denver, one of my friends trying
for a second child called me crying, saying she had gotten a
positive pregnancy test and began bleeding a week later. I
didn't have any words for her besides, "I'm so sorry." I didn't
understand the pain and hurt she was feeling. I didn't appreciate how it must feel to know that a life tried to start in you,
but wasn't able to make it. I didn't see the enormity in the
situation, because I felt it was such a brief amount of time
to have known she was pregnant. I was ignorant back then.

MONTH 8

I began hoping that maybe the eighth month would be
a charm. We had been married for almost a year, had a solid
and committed relationship, and financially we were able to
provide for a child.

I gave in and made copies of the fertility chart in the index section of the book I'd borrowed months before and dove in. There were multiple "problems" with my chart according to the book. I didn't notice any cervical mucus until day nineteen. The average day that a female ovulates is day fourteen, and I was *just* beginning to notice signs.

Also, even though I was taking my temperature every morning at the same time, my readings were all over the place. I also didn't get a positive OPK reading for any cycle days from day ten to eighteen, at which point I gave up testing.

I did observe a noticeable increase in temperature (an indication that ovulation has already occurred) around day twenty-eight, far from day fourteen. My cycle that month lasted thirty-nine days (a normal menstrual cycle is twenty-one to thirty-five days), a strong indicator that I had ovulated much later than normal.

To blow off steam, I went on a walk with my then thirty-six-year-old friend Katie. Katie and I met in graduate school where we spent many late nights not only studying for exams and writing papers together, but socializing at concerts, happy hours, and runs in the park. We both shared a love for international travel, and had spent three weeks traveling together in Vietnam. I considered her one of my best friends. She started dating her boyfriend close to the time of our wedding the year before and had very recently announced her engagement.

"I have something to tell you," she said.

I knew what was coming, and I braced myself.

"I'm pregnant, due next May," she said.

"Katie! That's wonderful!" I said. "Wow. That happened fast."

"Yeah, I know. We literally found out about a week after Jeff proposed," she said. "You know, I'm thirty-six, and I'm not getting any younger. It sucks that I'll be pregnant at the wedding, which is in November, by the way. But I'm glad it happened sooner rather than later, because of my age."

"I'm so happy for you," I said. And I was. Sort of. As thrilled as I was to hear her news, it was difficult because of our situation. I did my best to put aside my sob story long enough to congratulate her, but it wasn't long before I broke down and confessed what I was experiencing.

"We've been trying for eight months to get pregnant, and it just isn't happening," I said.

"That must be tough," she said. "But you're only thirty-two. You have plenty of time."

I understood that I was only in my early thirties, but I wasn't convinced that my age was helping our situation. The guilt I felt afterward for taking away Katie's special moment left me feeling ashamed, hoping more than ever for an end to my anguish.

5

DOUBTING MY FAITH

"To blame any misfortune on God, as if it could possibly be His will, is total ignorance. God's will for man and all creation is absolute good, and God cannot will or endorse sickness or limitation of any kind."
- John Randolph Price, *The Superbeings*

I did not consider myself religious, so I did not turn to any sort of faith to support me while attempting to get pregnant. I knew I believed in a higher power, but was confused about what that actually meant. I attended Mile Hi Church sporadically, but did not practice the teachings. If I did believe there was a God, I wondered what I could have done to be denied what I believed to be my natural right to bear children.

I began to doubt myself, and I wondered if I had somehow pissed off God, and He was responding by not allowing me to have a child. I wondered if this God judged me for past mistakes. I attempted to negotiate, saying that I would become a better person if I could just be blessed with a child. I didn't know how to pray, so I begged by closing my eyes and saying, "Please, PLEASE!" over and over again.

I was raised in the Lutheran faith until eighth grade when I decided enough was enough. As a young child, I remember attending Sunday school each week, and enjoying it. I liked the songs, I thought the teachers were kind, I had a lot of fun at Vacation Bible School, and I really liked the other kids in my class. As I got closer to adolescence, I began to question why my brother, mom, and I went to church each week, but my dad stayed home. I was an outspoken and opinionated child, so I asked my dad directly why he didn't attend with us. He replied that while he believed in God, Jesus, and the Bible, he had his "own way of worshipping." I found that to be an interesting statement, as I had never witnessed him reading the Bible and had never heard him discussing religion. My mom never got her driver's license, so my dad had to drive us all to church anyway, and he would pick us up after the service was over.

My mom took religion very seriously, to the point that I was often reminded that "God is watching you," and that I should "Honor thy father and thy mother." My mom felt it was important to attend Sunday school every single week, even though I eventually protested that I didn't enjoy it, and didn't want to go. She insisted that we attend, even going so far as dragging us out of bed to get ready for it. I was forced to take Catechism Class for a number of years, memorizing facts and taking tests. I became "confirmed" in eighth grade, but have never stepped foot in my childhood church after that day, except to attend the baptisms of my nephew and niece.

It wasn't until I lived in New Zealand that I became interested in religion again. My roommate mentioned a non-denominational church on the campus of Massey University in Auckland. The pastor was from Tennessee, and I liked how friendly and welcoming he was. I attended a few times with her but eventually became disenchanted with the idea. All the Jesus and bible talk and Christian rock music reminded me of the way religion had been forced upon me. I turned my back on organized religion, and moved on to my own form of spirituality instead.

Another roommate in New Zealand had left the book *Conversations with God Book I* by Neale Donald Walsch on our kitchen table. I picked it up, began reading, and found it hard to put down. The book was a different take on God than the one I had grown up with, and I found I could relate to what I was reading. This book was my introduction to spirituality—something I would embrace in the years to come.

One of the most difficult aspects to accept on this fertility journey was the number of people I knew or read about who were able to have kids who I believed shouldn't. I had strong opinions about the fairness of being allowed to have a child, and I wondered how it was possible for someone like Andrea Yates to be blessed with five children, only to drown them all in a bathtub. Or Susan Smith who drove her car into a lake and drowned her two young children. If there really was a God, how did He allow things like this to happen? I could not make sense of these incidents and felt something was being held against me. There are too many examples to count regarding children who are physically, emotionally, and mentally abused and neglected, along with those who are eventually murdered, and many who grow up to become hostile themselves. I was overwhelmed with the injustice of it all.

I even went so far as to question the financial aspect of raising children. I praised myself for not becoming pregnant at an age when I would not have been able to provide for a child. I patted myself on the back for achieving bachelor's and master's degrees by the time I was ready to have children. I was proud of my husband for getting a master's degree and starting his own consulting business. We had both traveled the world, and I felt we were able to financially provide for children. We had planned it out ahead of time, and we had acted like two responsible adults. I could not make sense of why couples who were struggling to pay their rent and bills were blessed with having three and four children. I was shocked at the teen pregnancy epidemic, the number of abortions that were performed, and the multitudes of drug addicts who conceived and gave birth to addicted babies. I judged all these people as undeserving. I never knew their full story, and I didn't care. I was angry, confused, disappointed, and outraged at what I considered the unfairness of it all.

6

ANOTHER YEAR OLDER

"Regardless of what you want to do or who you are, fear will always see you as wholly unqualified for anything you ever dream or attempt."
                                                                    - Jon Acuff

MONTH 9

I had taken a private practice class in graduate school teaching the fundamentals of starting a private psychotherapy practice. I decided opening a practice would be a good distraction from our attempts to conceive, and would provide extra income. My goal was eventually to move out of my full-time job into a private practice where I could set my own work hours and be my own boss. I referenced my class notes, sought out advice from established professionals, created a website, found office space, and prepared for a January 2010 opening.

Meanwhile, a friend referred me to an OB/GYN familiar with fertility issues. This OB had difficulty conceiving her second child. I thought she would be the perfect doctor to shed light on what might be occurring with my body. She advised me to schedule an appointment for day three of my menstrual cycle for accurate blood work results. I was relieved that she recognized the importance of the correct cycle day, unlike the doctor I'd had previously. I was again tested for luteinizing hormone (LH), follicle stimulating hormone (FSH), and estradiol, in addition to progesterone and testosterone (free and total). I assumed the progesterone test was performed to ensure I had ovulated and was not pregnant, and the testosterone tests were to rule out polycystic ovarian syndrome (PCOS).

All the test results were "normal." This time my LH was actually lower than my FSH, indicating I probably did not have PCOS. I wondered what was preventing me from becoming pregnant.

The doctor recommended a "semen analysis" for Patrick to rule out the possibility that he might be part of the perceived problem. I never doubted that the report would come back as anything other than normal, and I was correct.

"Patrick, I'm so sorry," I cried.

"Sorry for what?" he asked.

"It's obviously my fault this isn't working, but I can't figure out why."

"What do you mean it's your *fault*? Your hormone tests always come back normal. Even if there was something going on with you, I wouldn't consider it your *fault*!"

I allowed myself to feel grateful, at least that night, that even though we were struggling, Patrick was supportive. I felt reassured our marriage would survive this challenge.

October 1, 2009

After tonight's conversation with Patrick, I'm feeling more positive about things. I'm just one of thousands, actually millions of people who have issues with this. Hopefully this will be a short run and we'll be on our way to having a beautiful child. At the moment, my goal is to do everything I can to mentally take care of myself, and of course physically… This is a bump in the road, one of life's many challenges. By remaining positive and having hope, knowing that whatever is happening is supposed to, allowing life to flow as it should, I can get past it.

I had heard about a device called a fertility monitor— something that could help me determine when I ovulate based on the increasing LH. This hormone is always present in the urine and increases twenty-four to forty-eight hours prior to ovulation, the most fertile time of the cycle. The monitor I purchased claimed it had 99 percent accuracy in detecting the LH surge. I used this monitor in conjunction with ovulation predictor kit test strips, which also test for the LH surge. I was convinced that if somehow one of the methods didn't work, the other one would. The fertility monitor was more accurate than the ovulation kits, so I relied on it the most.

The fertility monitor had three readings of "low fertility," "high fertility," and "peak fertility." Peak fertility indicated ovulation would soon occur, and it was the ideal reading. According to my chart this month, I had a "high fertility" reading for thirteen days, beginning on day twelve of my cycle. Finally on day twenty-six, the monitor changed to "low fertility," indicating I more than likely did *not* ovulate. Also, I never got a positive confirmation on any of the OPKs indicating I was going to ovulate. This cycle was thirty-seven days in length. I now fit into the "irregular menstrual cycles" category.

I celebrated my thirty-third birthday on a chilly and rainy October night. We went out to dinner, but it was difficult to be festive, as it was another reminder of getting older and no closer to a baby.

November 9, 2009

…There is nothing to indicate that I ovulated this month, so here we go again…One of the things pointed out to me today was how my attitude toward this whole conception thing is one of defeat. Positive thinking is what's been lacking, and I've known that. I've just done nothing about it. It's time for an attitude adjustment. I'm over feeling sorry for myself. I'm going to be proactive and think positively. Things will happen as they should.

MONTH 10

I began researching reproductive endocrinologists (REs) in the Denver area. REs have extensive training on the endocrine system, and are more knowledgeable than OB/GYNs regarding fertility. I pulled out the Colorado Center for Reproductive Medicine (CCRM) referral that my general practitioner had given me six months prior, but quickly realized the facility did not accept my health insurance. I decided on another provider that was in network and made an appointment.

November 18, 2009

Dear Baby,

. . . As painful as it is knowing that I'm still not pregnant, I think I've put into place some things that might bring us closer to you. Today I'm beginning a liver cleanse recommended by an Ayurvedic holistic practitioner. He seems to think that the liver is connected to a lot of what I'm experiencing. Your dad and I also have an appointment scheduled for Friday with a fertility specialist. It hasn't been quite a year yet of trying, but by following my cycle closely I know that something is not quite right. So fingers crossed we get some answers and can move forward . . .

Love,

Mom

When I initially called to make the RE appointment, the office said the doctor who had been at the practice for many years was not available to meet with new patients. So I was assigned to a doctor who had just started. This unnerved me a bit, but I knew how rigorous the endocrinology medical training was and assumed I was in good hands.

Patrick and I went to the appointment together, and were impressed with the new RE. She was empathetic, patient, and intelligent, and took her time answering my many questions, despite our late Friday afternoon appointment time. We discussed medical history, the female reproductive system, and how to time intercourse. We also discussed having a hysterosalpingography (HSG), basically a dye test, to see if my fallopian tubes were clear. If the tubes were in any way blocked, it would show up on the test.

An ultrasound completed the visit. The RE noticed what appeared to be a fibroid on the outside of my uterus, but wasn't certain. She told me to come back when one of the ultrasonographers was available to take a closer look. She reassured me that my uterus looked normal.

I returned to the office three days later, which happened to be the first day of my menstrual cycle. Fortunately, they could still perform the ultrasound and HSG. The fibroid was still present, but they reassured me that it should not present a problem with getting pregnant because it was on the outside of the uterus. Additionally, the ultrasound revealed I had approximately twelve to thirteen follicles on each ovary, plenty to become pregnant. The HSG result was normal. While researching HSGs, I discovered conception rates increase after having one because the fallopian tubes get cleared out. I hoped it would be true for me.

I was instructed to take 50mg of Clomid, an ovulation-inducing drug taken orally, on day three of my cycle, and to take it for a total of five days, then come back to the office on day twelve to check for follicle development.

I returned to the office, where an ultrasound revealed that a few follicles had responded to the medication by growing larger. Also, my uterine lining was getting thicker, increasing the odds of implantation. I was told to use an OPK for the next few days and return for another ultrasound if a positive result was not detected.

I called the office four days later.

"I think I got a positive OPK result, but I can't be certain," I said. "The reference line is just slightly darker than my line."

"Come in and we'll do an ultrasound," the nurse said.

I returned for an ultrasound check, which revealed a dominant follicle of 19 millimeters. Most REs prefer follicle growth of 18–20 millimeters to proceed.

"Go ahead and inject Ovidrel tonight. This will force ovulation to occur," the nurse said. "Also, be sure to have sex for the next two days to cover the window."

I became frustrated with the inability to accurately detect if I was ovulating or not. How could I be taking a drug that should induce ovulation, but then take a test that couldn't tell me if it was happening? I recalled a friend who said she knows every month when she ovulates because she feels cramping on one side of her abdomen. Every month! I had never experienced that. I picked up the Ovidrel at the pharmacy and told my husband how to inject it because I was too afraid to do it myself.

Ten days after the injection, I got my period. This marked eleven months of unsuccessful attempts to create our baby. I was running out of patience. I began racking my brain for reasons it wasn't working. As various speculations swam around my head and I guessed I had everything from hormonal defects to cancer, I thought back to the time when I didn't own a computer, and when Google didn't exist. Information came from books. Research took time and effort, and I often was too lazy to do it. Not having immediate access to medical information allowed me to remain blissfully ignorant. I did not read a few articles and then diagnose myself with cancer or thyroid disease. And as unhappy as it made me, I still have trouble refraining from Google searching when a health concern arises.

We had an ugly sweater holiday party at our house to help lighten the mood. I looked forward to a good laugh. Not long into the party, my twenty-seven-year-old friend Ellie informed me she was pregnant. I had not told Ellie about our challenges, but she had shared with me that she had experienced many months without getting a period. Her pregnancy was a complete surprise. I reflected on the lesson I had learned in the way I reacted to Katie's pregnancy news three months prior, and decided to simply congratulate my friend. I couldn't help being envious, and noting how her age was on her side, especially if she wanted to have a second child.

Next Staci, my thirty-six-year-old friend announced her happy news. As thrilled as I was that she had been successful, I struggled to grasp why it wasn't happening for me and Patrick. I began to ruminate on how life just didn't seem fair.

MONTH 11

An acquaintance told me about a fertility drug called letrozole (trade name Femara), used primarily for breast cancer patients after surgery. However, it had been used off label since 2001 for ovarian stimulation because it was found to have lesser side effects than Clomid. My friend enumerated several friends of hers who had gotten pregnant while using this drug, so I suggested it to my RE. She agreed to prescribe 2.5 mg (the lowest dose) of letrozole to begin on day three of my cycle.

I was fortunate that my health insurance policy covered infertility testing, mostly because my RE billed the services under major medical due my fibroid cyst. My responsibility for the cost of the HSG a month prior at $568 was a bit higher than expected, but the out of pocket cost can be anywhere from $800 to $1,500 on average, so I considered myself lucky. I understood that my insurance would not cover assisted reproductive technologies (ART), such as intrauterine insemination (IUI) and in vitro fertilization (IVF).

December 25, 2009

Merry Xmas in L.A. where it's currently 75 degrees. I love the feel of the sun on my body. I'm convinced now more than ever that we need to live in a warmer state. I've loved CA from the day I first visited in 1996. I can see it in our future.

2010

I reported back to the RE office on January 2 of the New Year to check for follicle development. Unfortunately, this day fell on a Saturday, and I was not able to meet with my regular RE. Rather, I met with a doctor I was not entirely comfortable with, as our personalities didn't mesh. She performed an ultrasound and found a 21-millimeter follicle on my left ovary. This was 2 millimeters larger than the previous month, but I still wasn't aware of what the numbers meant at the time. I asked about the possibility of a luteal phase defect and asked if they could look at my progesterone level to determine if this was a problem. She asked me to schedule a progesterone level check for nine days out. I then asked her if there was anything I could do naturally to try to ovulate more regularly.

"How much do you exercise?" she asked.

"I work out four to five days a week for about an hour," I said. "I run anywhere from one to two and a half miles on the treadmill each day, and do strength training two to three days a week, along with crunches and lunges. I did run a marathon, but that was four years ago."

"That's quite a bit of exercise," she stated. "I recommend decreasing your workouts and increasing your dietary fat intake."

"How do you mean?" I asked.

"Try eating more ice cream," she suggested.

This doctor explained that it usually takes pretty drastic changes in exercise regimens to affect a change in ovulation. She then explained it was possible that I had "idiopathic ovulation dysfunction," or failure of my ovaries to release an egg. When I looked at her chart notes, I saw she had actually written "idio*pathetic*." How ironic!

"It can take some time to conceive even after ovulation is established," the doctor added. "I think you should consider IUIs as a next step. And remember, you need to use the Ovidrel tonight to trigger ovulation."

When I returned home, I Googled the definition of "excessive exercise," and concluded I did not fit the description. I also took into consideration my weight at the time of 117 pounds and height of five feet one, and came up with a body mass index of 22.1, which fell into the middle of the "normal" category.

My progesterone bloodwork result indicated I had indeed ovulated that month. I had been tracking my temperature, and a few days after I received this result, my temperature dropped. I understood this was an indication that progesterone levels were beginning to drop, and I should expect my period to arrive in the next week or so. I called the office to notify them of the drop in temperature, and scheduled a consult with my doctor to discuss next steps.

In the meantime, I sought out a naturopathic medical facility, focusing on hormonal concerns. I was pleased with what I read about the primary doctor, and hoped she could get to the bottom of what might be going on with my body. Despite all my blood work coming back normal, I knew my body better than anyone else did, and I knew something wasn't right. So I proceeded with the appointment. This doctor took a thorough evaluation of my health history, and instructed me to come back for blood work as soon as my cycle ended.

7

A New Year

"If we bring a symbolic attitude to our lives, searching out the meaning of what happens to us and thereby allowing our own capacity to make wholeness out of the random and disparate events of our lives, then no matter what happens in the plot, whatever the setting, whoever the characters, major and minor, we will see that indeed, there are no accidents in the stories of our lives."

- Robert H. Hopcke

A few days after the naturopathic consultation, Patrick and I met again with the RE.

"So what can I help you with today?" she asked.

"I've been tracking my temperature, and it dropped two days ago. Last month when it dropped, I got my period a few days later."

"But you haven't gotten your period yet?" she asked.

"No, but I can feel the symptoms. It's going to arrive any day now. What would you advise trying next?"

"Have you taken a pregnancy test?"

"No way. I've been disappointed too many times by the negative result, that I just can't bear another one."

"The fact that you haven't gotten your period yet is positive though," she said.

"Yes, but I'm sure it will come soon. I am having a difficult time with all of this," I confessed. "Even though my cycles have regulated with the medication, I keep wondering why I haven't become pregnant. I can't stop thinking about all of this, and as time goes on, I get more and more stressed. I understand there's probably a correlation between stress and fertility, so I know it doesn't help."

"The fact that you haven't conceived yet is not out of the ordinary, and doesn't concern me. You haven't been trying for a year yet, and you've only been with our facility for a few months," she explained.

"I hear you, and believe me, I feel pathetic," I said. "I have always been a goal setter, and for the most part, have always completed those goals. My life plan included having children, and I feel like I'm slipping further away from that."

"I am going to refer you to a psychologist who we work with regularly. She is very familiar with the negative impact fertility issues can have on a person, and can demonstrate mind-body techniques to help reduce your stress and help you better cope with your attempts to get pregnant. I suggest making an appointment."

"I will do that. Thanks. I also don't think I'm ready to try an IUI yet, but I'll let you know if I change my mind," I said. "If I don't get pregnant next month, maybe I'll be ready for one."

"That sounds like a plan," she said. "Please call us if you don't get your period so we can do a pregnancy test."

I felt ashamed as I left the office. I was emotionally out

of control, and I did not possess the coping skills or tools to manage my anxiety. I felt like a failure, both to myself and to my husband. I was distraught that my body provided such a healthy temple for so long, and when I wanted it to do what so many women could do naturally, even by accident, I was not succeeding. I realized I had a perfectionistic personality, something I had possibly been living with my entire life. I was not able to accept that I was not succeeding at getting pregnant. It affected all areas of my life: sleep, work, marriage, friendships, etc. The really concerning part was that we had not even tried for a year yet. I didn't realize how much I relied on success to feed my self-esteem and confidence. For so many years as a child, I was told how imperfect I was, and I felt my inability to conceive simply proved it.

I was unable to accept this wasn't happening, and found it difficult to think about anything else. Despite being a professional counselor, I was unable to reason with myself. I knew how I would counsel others going through something similar, but I could not counsel myself.

I scheduled an appointment with the psychologist recommended by my RE. I explained what a difficult time I was having trying to conceive, and she empathized with my challenge. Some of the pressure I had been feeling began to lift after that appointment. I knew I was moving in a positive direction.

8

THAT SECOND LINE

"Every great work, every big accomplishment, has been brought into manifestation through holding to the vision, and often just before the big achievement comes apparent failure and discouragement."
                                                    - Florence Scovel Shinn

On January 19, 2010, four days after I met with the RE, I took a home pregnancy test. Patrick was working in Charlotte, North Carolina, but I decided to take the test anyway. I set the test down and walked away, not wanting to be disappointed when the second line did not appear. I held my breath as I waited at least four minutes to go back and check on it. When I went back to the bathroom, there it was: that second line I had been waiting almost a year to see—347 days to be exact. I called the fertility clinic on my way to work, stating that I had a positive home test, and they had me come in for a human chorionic gonadotropin (hCG) and progesterone blood draw.

At work that day, I wasn't able to concentrate on anything but the results of those tests. I stared at my phone on and off for the next three hours, when it finally rang. My RE personally called to reveal that I was indeed pregnant, with an hCG level of 494 (a level of 50 or above indicates a viable pregnancy) and a progesterone level of 30 (a level of 20 or above produces the best ongoing pregnancy outcomes). She congratulated me and instructed me to come back in three days to re-test the hCG level. I called my husband right away. "I'm pregnant!" I screamed.

"We did it!" he said.

Hearing his excitement meant the world to me, and I couldn't wait for him to return from his trip. For the rest of the work day, I felt like I was in a dream, as if I were floating on air. I walked down the hall to my colleague's office to tell her the good news. She was one of the few people I had shared our fertility journey with, and she gave me my first congratulatory hug.

January 19, 2010

Dear Baby,

I'm so happy to report that the wait is finally over! I can't explain the joy and relief I felt today. I started getting excited and thinking about what we will name you, and how we will tell your grandparents, but then had to remind myself that things can go wrong in the first three months of a pregnancy. So I know

I need to slow down and take things day by day. I'm over the moon that you decided to join us in this life, and I can't wait to meet you! Fingers crossed that everything continues to go smoothly. Words can't explain how grateful I feel, and how much I'm looking forward to being your mother.

Love,

Mom

I learned it is very important to get a second hCG reading, because the first one above 50 does not tell you anything besides you are probably pregnant. Ideally, this number should double within forty-eight hours, or should at least rise by 60 percent. I knew nothing about this at the time, and assumed everything would be fine. My repeat blood draw was seventy-two hours later, and the result was 1,685, more than tripling in this time frame. I was told that I was indeed pregnant, but needed to schedule an OB appointment with my doctor for an ultrasound to ensure it was a viable pregnancy.

During this visit, I was informed of ectopic pregnancies and cautions, and was reminded that my blood type was Rh negative. Because of my A negative blood type, I was told to call the office if I had any bright red bleeding because I might need the RhoGAM shot. I did not understand what this meant and hoped I would not need the shot. I went home with my ectopic pregnancy precautions and Googled what that meant, and of course, I became concerned that it might happen to me.

My next appointment was an ultrasound about two weeks after the initial positive hCG result. I found out I was six weeks and three days pregnant, and my due date was September 25, 2010. I was pregnant with one baby only, and the baby's heartbeat was 114 beats per minute.

"Don't tell us the gender, please!" Patrick said. "We don't want to know!"

"Well, that won't be a problem," the ultrasound technician said. "We can't possibly know that until at least a few weeks from now!" She laughed.

About two weeks later, I was sitting on our basement couch when I felt a twinging feeling in my abdomen. It would come and go, but seemed to last for some time. I became agitated, and I contacted the office to let them know. I described the feeling as a "pinching sensation." I wondered if I was going to go down in history as their most anxious patient to date. At that stage of my life, I hate to admit that I didn't care. We had worked hard to achieve this pregnancy, and I wasn't taking any chances.

I went for my second ultrasound to ensure things were progressing smoothly with the pregnancy due to the uterine pinching sensations. The clinical note stated:

"Jennifer comes in today complaining of pelvic 'twinging.' She states that the pains are rapid in onsets and resolve quickly, but are concerning since she has never had them before. She is currently 8 weeks 3 days gestation dated by the day of her hCG trigger shot. Today's ultrasound revealed a single intrauterine pregnancy with good fetal cardiac activity. The amnion was clearly identified surrounding the fetus. The crown-rump length measured 1.94 cm, which is consistent with an 8 week 2 day gestation. There has been appropriate interval growth since her last ultrasound." I began to empathize with health insurance companies at this point. This was a good example of why they cover only a few ultrasounds during pregnancy, or people like me would be in every week! I then remembered my monthly insurance premium increase, and I didn't feel as sorry for them.

I had my first OB/GYN appointment a few weeks later and began to relax. By this time, we had revealed the wonderful news to a small number of our close friends, as well as Patrick's family. We decided to notify my family in person with a visit to Chicago when I would be about twelve weeks along. When we told them about the pregnancy, it never occurred to me to tell them to keep it a secret. According to everything I had read, twelve weeks was the crossover point into the safe zone. My doctor had mentioned that miscarriage rates drastically drop after the first trimester, and I was just about done with trimester one.

When I was nineteen weeks pregnant, we traveled to Kauai, Hawaii and met up with Sandy and Pat, my in-laws. It was the first time we had seen them in person since announcing the news. Sandy ran up to us at the airport, gave us a big bear hug, and exclaimed "We're so excited for you!" Patrick's parents did not have any grandchildren yet. Our baby would be their first, and it was clear how they felt about it!

We rented a car and toured around the small island, visiting the breathtaking Waimea Canyon and the secluded Polihale Beach. We kayaked the Wailua River and hiked through a forest to the Uluwehi Falls.

"I'm impressed you guys are so adventurous," I said to my in-laws. "There's no way my parents would have gone on a trip like this. Thanks for making the effort!"

"We're impressed with YOU, Jen. You're the one who's almost five months pregnant!"

"Well, I'm glad we're able to take such a fabulous 'baby-moon.' Traveling will become a bit more complicated once baby arrives!" I said.

Around twenty weeks into my pregnancy, I transferred from my OB to a midwifery practice at a major hospital in Colorado. I felt my OB was too "Western-minded" for my taste and preferred to work with a group I hoped would be more "alternative or Eastern-minded." I also Googled a bit of information regarding C-section rates at a handful of local Colorado hospitals, and discovered the hospital my OB used had the highest C-section rate.

I researched "water births," and decided I liked what I read about this method. Only a few facilities in Colorado offer this type of birth, and the hospital I ended up choosing was not only on board with water births, but had a lower rate of C-sections. After making the water birth decision, I periodically second-guessed my ability to labor and deliver in a tub without medication or an epidural, but believed I could be strong enough to do it. My friend had delivered her baby without any medication, solely because she is afraid of the epidural needle. I once asked her to rate the pain level on a scale of one to ten. She said seven. When I pressed her for the true number, she said, "Okay, probably an eight." I wondered if she was still downplaying it, and if it was more likely a nine or a ten!

The midwife team of four consisted of three what I would call "younger" ladies, and one "senior" lady. They were all friendly and took their time answering my numerous questions, but I discovered their views were not far off from my former OB. I suppose this is because they worked for, and were trained in, a major, nationally recognized hospital. However, I was certain I was in capable hands.

The twenty week ultrasound revealed a normally developing baby, and we were relieved. We proudly walked out with the grainy black and white photos that I planned on putting into the baby book I had purchased weeks earlier.

It was around this time in the pregnancy that I researched hypnobirthing. According to www.hypnobirthing.com, the Mongan Method Hypnobirthing, or hypnobirthing for short, is a "simple, straightforward program, thoughtfully developed over the years to remind mothers of the simplicity of birth itself. Just as the majority of birthing women do not need interventions and procedures for a safe and healthy birth, they do not need a complex set of exercises and scripts to prepare themselves for peaceful, calm and comfortable birthing. The birthing body and the baby know just what to do. Mongan Method HypnoBirthing® is designed to teach women to trust in Nature's way of birth and to relax and let their bodies do what is needed. By practicing a few key techniques, mothers program their minds and condition their bodies to birth easily. When it comes to programming and conditioning, variety is not necessarily a good thing. Repetition is what gets the best result."

One of my work colleagues, a former nurse, was a certified hypnobirthing trainer and had nothing but positive things to say about this method. I also remember asking her about the physical side of labor. "How much did it hurt? Was it just in the abdomen? Was it tolerable?" She assured me it was more of a chronic pain than acute, that it was manageable, and that I'd do just fine, especially if I followed the hypnobirthing method! I went straight home and Googled hypnobirthing classes in my area, eventually settling on a nearby class that both my husband and I would be able to attend.

A number of my pregnant friends were opting to use doulas to assist with their births, so I Googled doulas as well. I learned that when doulas attend birth, labors are shorter with fewer complications. Babies are healthier, and they tend to breastfeed more easily. The instructor of our hypnobirthing class just happened to be a doula too. Patrick and I met up with her at a coffee shop, interviewed her with a million questions, and decided she would be a fantastic fit. We signed up for her five-week class and asked her to be our doula.

About twenty-eight weeks into the pregnancy, I tested positive for gestational diabetes, which I found odd, and wasn't quite able to accept. I went home and Googled gestational diabetes, and learned that only 4 percent of women actually experience this, and I did not fit into any of the risk categories. I recalled the nurse saying it was okay to eat before the test, so I had my almond butter and bread in the car on the way to the hospital. When the positive test came back, I mentioned that I had eaten before, and a different nurse said I should have fasted. I was brought in again to do a much longer test to determine if I did, indeed, have gestational diabetes, and the subsequent test came back normal.

In the course of our five-week hypnobirthing class, I learned about the Group B strep test, and how beneficial it would be to test negative for it. Group B streptococcus (strep), as it is known, is a bacteria carried in the intestines or lower genital tract, and approximately 25 percent of women test positive for it. Most babies born to women carrying strep are healthy, but the few who are infected during labor can become critically ill. I was informed that if I tested positive for it, I would be required to have continuous antibiotics throughout labor. Antibiotic therapy has risks, including allergic reactions, increased incidence of yeast infections and thrush, as well as encouraging penicillin-resistant strains of strep and other bacteria such as E. coli.

Our hypnobirthing instructor recommended probiotics for weeks before I would be taking the test. I did as instructed, but the test came back positive. My midwife convinced me that taking precaution during labor (i.e., using the antibiotics) could save the life of my baby. She went on to explain a few cases where this type of situation turned deadly, and I decided to follow her recommendations. This is just one example of a more Western-minded approach, despite what some might think about the way midwives practice.

At seven and a half months pregnant, I had become bigger and more exhausted. However, the adventure lover in me convinced Patrick that we should attend a friend's wedding in Big Sky, Montana. Instead of flying, I thought it would be a fun idea to take a twenty-four hour road trip. I even planned a few adventures along the way, such as an overnight stay in a teepee in Cody, Wyoming. We slept on an air mattress after a seven-and-a-half-hour drive. The fun didn't stop there. The next day, we drove through Yellowstone National Park and viewed the famous Old Faithful Geyser. We made it in time for the rehearsal dinner, where I am proud to say I whooped it up on the square-dancing floor. The twelve-hour drive back home was exhausting, and I spent most of the time sleeping in the back seat while Patrick listened to a book on CD.

At the end of August, we had a baby shower where we asked guests to predict the baby's gender and due date. Most people guessed our baby was a boy, and most assumed he or she would be born within a two-week time frame (a week before the due date to a week after), with a range from September 18 to October 3, 2010. I planned on working as far into the pregnancy as possible, which meant until September 17, 2010, eight days before the due date. I was convinced for some reason that this baby would arrive about a week earlier than the due date.

One of the hypnobirthing exercises required me to write a "Birth Story Wish," based on the way I hoped to experience the birth of my baby. Although I understood the birth would not go exactly the way I imagined, I believed storing a positive image in my memory could only enhance the birth experience. I wrote:

"I feel relaxed and peaceful leading up to the first surges (contractions) because I took the time to practice self-care. As I feel the first surges, I remain calm and begin practicing the breathing techniques I learned. I visualize how exciting it will be to meet my new baby. I continue to relax for as long as possible. Once I feel the need, I take a warm, relaxing bath. I keep my eyes closed, and continue to go within myself. When it is time to move to the birth center (hospital), I calmly dry myself off and change into comfortable clothing. There is very light traffic on the way, and the car ride is smooth. Patrick is nervous, but excited that he will meet his daughter or son soon! The hospital staff greets me with warm and gentle smiles, and the check-in process goes smoothly. I am led to a dimly lit room where the birthing tub has been set up. Throughout the next few hours, I listen to music, work with the exercise ball, practice breathing, and labor in the tub. The water takes away the discomfort I was feeling, and I know that the birth of my baby is going to happen very soon. Active labor has lasted less than 10 hours, and my baby is put on my chest by Patrick. The baby is easily able to latch on and feed. The baby weighs less than 8 pounds and is perfectly healthy. The baby continues to feed regularly, and it is eventually time to introduce the baby to our home."

My sister-in-law had given me advice a few months prior, recommending I "just be open to whatever happens." I believe this was in response to me declaring that I knew it would never get to the point that I would need a C-section. Maybe I wouldn't complete an actual water birth, and I might elect to get the epidural, but a C-section? I didn't think so.

My labor and birth went nothing like I expected or planned, and was nowhere near my Birth Story Wish. To summarize, at almost forty-two weeks of pregnancy, my midwife ruptured my membranes to avoid having to induce me in the hospital. It was unpleasant, and I have since questioned the decision, but it started things moving. However, I didn't experience that gush of water I had witnessed so often in TV shows and movies. Slight contractions started about thirty-six hours later, eventually becoming closer together and more and more painful. After debilitating back labor, we made the uncomfortable drive to the hospital. I was immediately hooked up to a monitor and was told I was dilated only 2 centimeters. For real?

Everything went downhill from there. I never got off the monitor (I had planned to walk around, use the stability ball, etc.), the birthing tub never made it to my room, I got an epidural, and I never made it past 6-centimeter dilation. On numerous occasions, a team of doctors and nurses rushed in to give me oxygen after having a long contraction. I became frightened at the direction things were going. I was told I could try for a vaginal delivery, but the possibility of an emergency situation was real at this point. I eventually began experiencing the dreaded back labor again, even with the epidural.

I looked up at the clock, which read 4:45 p.m. It was October 9, 2010. If I lasted another seven hours or so, my baby would be born on 10/10/10. Not only would that be exciting, but it was also my dad's birthday. After considering safety and my utter exhaustion, my husband and I opted for the C-section. My doula tried to encourage me to stick it out, but said I needed to do what was best for the baby and me. She complemented me on my hypnobirthing breathing techniques. I apologized to her for not being strong enough to deliver naturally, bursting into tears, as my childhood trauma of never feeling good enough came flooding back. She and Patrick supported me emotionally the best they could, while I struggled to accept the reason for the C-section—fetal distress—and off we went to the operating room. I later learned that my baby had the cord wrapped around his neck twice!

At 6:55 p.m. on October 9, 2010, Liam Walter Noonan was born. I will never forget hearing him cry for the first time, pausing long enough to hear me say, "Hi, baby boy. I'm so glad you're here!" I was convinced he had recognized my voice, and it made everything we just went through completely worth it.

My mother-in-law flew in from California to help us for a week. I was humbled that she stepped up to the plate, knowing that my own mom would not. Watching her hold and caress her first grandchild was a beautiful site, and I was so grateful for her support.

After comparing my actual birth process to my Birth Story Wish, I humbly grasped a very tough and important lesson: to embrace the unknown. This allowed me to consider all the times in my life when I attempted to control an outcome before it happened. From a young age, I felt as if I needed to take control of my life, because it felt out of control. I did not feel I was being properly supported at home, and therefore I felt I needed to support myself. I thought if I allowed enough time to plan, and put a solid plan into place, things would turn out close to the way I hoped. This turned out to be the case on many occasions. However, the stress and anxiety I experienced along the way were not conducive to my overall health. I believe this was one of the reasons it took 347 days to get a positive pregnancy test. I learned the hard lesson that life cannot be controlled.

9

A NEW DIRECTION

"Your environment is always changing. If you shift your focus from allowing your external environment to elicit a state of joy or a feeling of joy and you consciously decide to be joyous regardless of any situation then you will have a joyful life. If you choose joy moment to moment then you will have a life of joy."

- Danielle Rama Hoffman

A few months into maternity leave, I informed my employer that I would not be returning to my position. I wanted to spend as much time as possible with Liam, and Patrick and I had come to the conclusion that we could make it work financially. I began seeing clients in my private practice again when Liam was just six weeks old. Patrick continued to work on his real estate venture and was working from home, so he was able to watch Liam while I was at work.

When I wasn't working, Liam and I strolled around the neighborhood admiring the dazzling fall colors. I took an enormous number of photos of him, believing everything he did, and especially the way he smiled, was exquisite. I filled up photo book after photo book with these pictures, and spent many hours on his baby book and scrapbooks. I laughed at his cooing, babbling, and squealing.

In contrast, I cried when I didn't know how to soothe him. I worried when he was gaining weight and height so slowly and wouldn't drink as much breast milk as the pediatrician said he should. I agonized over how little homemade baby food he ate, which I had spent so much time making. I was well aware of how blessed we were to have Liam but couldn't help thinking how getting what you want doesn't always lead to a trouble-free life.

A few months later, Patrick was asked to be part of a team of consultants for an eight-month geographic information systems project in the Inland Empire area of California, a forty-five-minute drive east of Los Angeles. The downside was that he would be traveling back and forth each week. I enlisted the help of a friend to watch Liam while I met with clients when Patrick was traveling.

When Liam was just over five months old, Patrick and I discussed the possibility of moving to California, so the family could be together every day. Over the years, I had traveled to Lake Tahoe, San Francisco, Santa Cruz, Newport Beach, Venice, Santa Monica, Carlsbad, La Jolla, and San Diego, and I had fond memories of all my visits there. The fact that my in-laws already lived in southern California was a bonus, as they would have the pleasure of seeing their grandson grow up and maybe even help us with Liam from time to time.

The California work opportunity also gave us the financial freedom to begin planning a second-story addition to our home while we were away. We lived in a one-story brick bungalow with two bedrooms and a basement, and the addition would provide an extra bedroom for a second child. We decided to spend approximately eight months living in California, and return to our expanded home at the conclusion of the contract.

Before we left, I had to find a new health insurance plan. My former employer had switched to a Colorado-specific health insurance company the year my son was born, due to rising health care costs. The plan expired at the end of my maternity leave, which was the end of 2010. I decided to apply to be added to Patrick and Liam's plan. I answered the underwriting questions honestly and was rejected for abnormal platelet levels, having a fibroid, and having had moles removed. As healthy as I thought I was, the insurance company did not agree.

I then applied for an individual health plan with another insurance company. I disclosed my involvement with the reproductive endocrinology office, and received a rejection letter in the mail:

"We regret to inform you that your application for enrollment has been denied. Your application was not accepted due to: Treatment of infertility within the past 2 years."

I became discouraged and wondered how I was going to secure health insurance. I was fully aware of the ramifications of not having at least catastrophic coverage, and I began to panic. I decided to appeal the decision by writing a letter of my own, and pleading with my former reproductive endocrinologist to write a letter on my behalf. She did, and I was finally granted health insurance. The fight to secure it, and being denied due to infertility reasons, was traumatizing. However, I reminded myself that we were over the hurdle of conceiving and decided to be grateful instead of angry.

10

CALIFORNIA

"Inner faith can produce the people and events that you need; it will work. Even after you develop this faith in God and yourself, you will find that there still are obstacles in life."

- Dr. Wayne W. Dyer

The day finally arrived to drive our U-Haul to California with Liam, who was by then seven-and-a-half months old. With stops in Green River, Utah, and Las Vegas, Nevada, we arrived in Santa Monica where we lived for a month at my brother-in-law's bungalow while he was in Germany. I enjoyed the Santa Monica lifestyle, taking endless stroller walks to the beach, Third Street Mall, Farmer's Markets, and Montana Street.

We soon relocated to Claremont, a college town located approximately thirty miles east of Los Angeles in the Inland Empire. Claremont has approximately 35,000 residents and is known as "the city of trees and PhDs" due to the large number of trees and residents with doctoral degrees. We moved into a two-bedroom, one-bathroom apartment, which was a significant decrease in square footage from our home in Denver.

Claremont was a pleasant place to live. There really were a significant number of trees that bloomed beautifully at various times of the year, and "the Village" was full of fun shops and restaurants to explore. A train carrying commuters to and from Los Angeles and San Bernardino ran very close to our apartment. It took me a while to become used to the blaring horns late at night, but I got used to it.

The challenging part about living in California was that I did not know anyone in the area, and Patrick worked full time. The possibility of working as a counselor was out of the question. Although I was a licensed professional counselor in Colorado, there was no "reciprocity" among states. I was not legally able to practice counseling in California, unless I wanted to spend another few years accruing additional clinical hours to meet the state's requirements. We planned to live in California temporarily, so this was something I did not consider.

I joined a mom's group, and became good friends with one of the ladies with a son very close in age to Liam. Despite multiple outings scheduled each week, it was a lonely and isolating existence, and I became increasingly sad. Although my in-laws lived in the Los Angeles area, it was an hour to drive to their house. It would have been ideal to live close to them simply for some company, but unfortunately this was not the case. Patrick and I managed to visit them on weekends about once a month.

I made the decision to stop breastfeeding when Liam was nine months old because he was gaining weight more slowly than other babies his age. His California pediatrician recommended a blood growth hormone test. I became anxious that this was due to a lack of fat in my breast milk, so I switched him to formula. Not only did this not help, it caused a lot of constipation, which was even worse. I never followed up with the growth hormone test, hoping things would soon change.

Another reason for ceasing breastfeeding was the desire to try for a second child. I was approaching thirty-five, which would put me in the advanced maternal age category. I was concerned not only about our ability to conceive again, but the possibility of chromosomal abnormalities if we did. I had not had a period since the month we had conceived Liam, about nineteen months prior. I was aware of many stories of women getting their periods back soon after delivery, while most seemed to get it back within six months. Many were getting pregnant without a period while breastfeeding, because they simply had no idea when they were ovulating! I was not one of them. I waited and waited for my period to arrive so Patrick and I could consider trying to conceive a second child.

Eleven months after Liam's birth, my period arrived. I had a thirty-three-day cycle, so I believed my cycles had normalized. Maybe my body knew what it was doing now, and I would have an easy time getting pregnant this time, I thought.

Patrick and I officially decided to begin trying for a second child. Given what we had experienced the first time around, we were unsure how long it might take. Also, the original plan was that Liam and I would move back to Colorado toward the beginning of the year 2012, and Patrick would split his time between Colorado and California. That meant he would be 1,000 miles away four days of the week, every week, making it even harder to time our efforts to conceive.

The following month's cycle lasted forty-one long days. I became concerned that things hadn't normalized after all. I began researching reproductive endocrinologists in southern California. I may have been getting ahead of myself, but I was determined not to have a repeat of last time.

The reproductive facility we chose to work with was a thirty-minute drive from our apartment. I met with a warm and friendly female doctor, and I felt excited to work with her. She ordered the standard battery of blood tests and told me to make an appointment to discuss the results. Before we could meet, I received a letter stating that the doctor I had met with was leaving the practice, and I was being reassigned.

I found that out over the Christmas holiday, and we were set to take a coastal road trip up to Big Sur. I had hoped to pick up the medication before we left, but the reproductive facility would not call in the prescription until it received my blood work results. Because my doctor had left, and her nurse was reassigned also, I was reduced to leaving voicemails, pleading for someone to call me back. By this time, I had received my results directly from the lab and knew they were normal. The office was closed New Year's Eve and New Year's Day, so we left on our road trip without the prescription.

New Year's Day 2012, we set out on our Central Coast road trip. We stopped in Solvang, a Danish village located in the heart of Santa Barbara wine country near the Santa Ynez Mountains, then headed to the coast, stopping in Morro Bay for lunch and to view the Morro Rock, a five-hundred-and-eighty-one-foot volcanic landform. We roamed around the quaint coastal town of Cayucos, and drove our car on the long stretches of golden sand on Pismo Beach.

Liam was almost fifteen months old and was an active little toddler. His blonde hair, striking blue eyes, and long eyelashes consistently captured the attention of strangers. So did his activity level! He had inherited my strong-willed and curious nature and was into just about everything. He was excited to explore the coast with us, and barely slept to avoid missing anything!

We soon made it to the coastal town of Cambria. We stayed for a few nights, going for long walks along the Pacific Ocean, taking in the spectacular scenery. I received a return call from one of the nurses at the reproductive facility, who called in a letrozole prescription to a pharmacy in Morro Bay, about a thirty-minute drive from where we had just been. After Liam fell asleep for the night, I headed back down the coast. Before the pharmacist handed the prescription to me, she looked at it quizzically, and almost alarmingly.

"You realize what this medication is for, correct?" she asked.

"Yes. I'm aware that it's a drug for breast cancer patients. I'm using it to induce ovulation to become pregnant," I confidently stated.

"Really? Okay, because it doesn't say that it should be used for that reason," she said.

"I know. I got pregnant with my son by using it, and I

know others who have as well," I responded.

"One of my friends is having trouble getting pregnant. I'll have to tell her about this," she said.

"I'm telling you, it works," I said, feeling happy I was able to spread some fertility cheer.

The next day, I took my first dose of letrozole. My last menstrual cycle lasted thirty-seven days, a few days past the normal range, so I assumed I was once again experiencing late ovulation. I viewed my decision to contact the California reproductive facility as a wise one.

Our road trip took us farther north up the coast to Hearst Castle, with a stop to see a colony of sea lions resting and playing. We traveled all the way through Big Sur to a cabin in the woods, halfway between the little town of Big Sur and Carmel. It was an ideal base for exploring the magnificent beauty of the two towns, as well as Pebble Beach,17 Mile Drive, and Monterey, where we visited the city's world-famous aquarium. We then drove back down the coast and across to Paso Robles. We took Liam to a park and ate at a delicious restaurant called Thomas Hill Organics. I recall this trip being one of our most scenic, and I remember how much hope I had that we would soon be adding to our family.

When we returned, I scheduled an ultrasound appointment with the reproductive facility. I looked forward to seeing the follicle development, hoping for adequate growth. I met with the doctor who had replaced my doctor, and discussed my reasons for trying letrozole again. He looked over my blood work and agreed with the plan. We moved to the ultrasound room, taking a close look at follicular development.

"Hmmm. Are you sure you haven't ovulated already?" he asked.

"I wouldn't think so. It's day eleven. I've never ovulated this early in a cycle. Why? What do you see?"

"Well, the size of the follicles indicates either you already ovulated or you're not even close."

"How would I know for certain?" I asked.

"A blood progesterone test would confirm it one way or the other. If you didn't ovulate, you could come back for another ultrasound to check for follicular development again."

"I'll have to think about it. My health insurance doesn't cover any of this, and I'm fairly certain I didn't ovulate." I understood that if I did the blood work and ultrasound, it would be $350 or so.

I left the office disappointed and confused, with racing thoughts. *I couldn't have ovulated this early, could I? If I did, we better have sex tonight just in case. And if I did, I would expect to get my period within the next ten days or so. That would mean a cycle length of twenty-one days, which would be very out of the ordinary. There's no way to be sure if I did besides paying hundreds of dollars. Do I want to do that knowing I most likely did not ovulate? Or should I simply watch for signs of ovulation, and make sure we continue to cover our bases?*

Trying to conceive a baby can take a huge toll on mental well-being. Most often, the one trying to physically get pregnant takes on the brunt of the worrying. I did not have a job to distract me, so I pondered these questions throughout the day—all day if I allowed it. Each day when Patrick came home from work, I would sit him down, make sure I had his full attention, and then unload all the information I had learned, and how I thought we should proceed. I am blessed to have a husband who is even-keeled and patient. Although he might have felt I was rambling on, and that we were going to proceed with my plan no questions asked, he remained empathetic through it all.

"Jen, I know you've done a lot of research. You know more about this than I do. It all sounds fine to me," he would say time and time again. "I know it's going to happen. I'm not concerned."

I admired his strength and positive attitude, but unfortunately it did not rub off on me. When cycle day twenty-one came and went, I was convinced I had not ovulated. I was curious if I was about to, or perhaps had in the last few days, but was not willing to pay $350 to confirm it, despite my husband's work contract extension.

By cycle day twenty-nine, I noticed some signs of ovulation, which I thought was strange. That would mean I wouldn't get my period until at least day thirty-nine or forty. As the days went on, I became increasingly frustrated, refusing to take a pregnancy test. I was well-aware of the disappointment that came with a negative result, and I knew long cycles had become typical for me.

Close to forty-five days into my cycle, I relented. I snuck to the bathroom early one morning and took a pregnancy test. As usual, I put the test on the bathroom counter without looking at it for some time, anticipating a negative result. I took a peek before I walked out of the bathroom and was shocked to see two pink lines.

"What? Oh my God! Patrick?"

"Yeah?"

"You won't believe this. I'm pregnant. The stick says I'm pregnant!"

"Really? That's fantastic!"

"I don't know how it happened. I have no idea when I ovulated, but it must have been late based on the signs I noticed. I guess it doesn't matter."

According to my last missed period, I was probably six weeks pregnant by that point. I researched a few OBs in the area, decided on one who received high reviews, and called. I made an appointment for a date when I would be close to eight or nine weeks along, when a heartbeat should be detectable.

I was shocked, but relieved, that we had achieved a pregnancy with the first round of medication. We decided to celebrate at Disney Land. Standing in line for the Tower of Terror at the nearby California Adventure Park, I put my hand on the slight bulge in my belly, and silently thanked my higher power. Liam was just sixteen months old, which would mean this baby would be born right after he turned two.

Although I knew it would be challenging to care for a toddler and a newborn back home in Denver while Patrick traveled to California each week, I was relieved we wouldn't have to endure months of trying to conceive like the last time. I also thought it was pretty spectacular that we had conceived our second child the same time of year we did our first!

At the beginning of March, we took a six-hour road trip east to Phoenix to spend a long weekend with my Aunt Cindy (my mom's sister) and her husband. It had been many years since I last saw my aunt, so it was wonderful catching up and going to the Colorado Rockies Spring Training baseball game. My Uncle Mike (my mom's brother) made a last-minute decision to drive up from Tucson. Although we had exchanged letters and emails, I had never met him in person.

I decided not to mention that I was pregnant. It was still early on, and I didn't want too many people to know before I'd crossed the first trimester threshold. I agreed to the wine that was offered with dinner, knowing Patrick would drink it for me while no one was looking.

"You and my mom are six years apart in age, right?" I asked my aunt.

"We are. From what I understand, my mom had a miscarriage after she had your mom, and I guess it took a while longer to get pregnant with me."

"Grandma had a miscarriage?" I said. "My mom never told me that."

"Maybe she didn't know. It wasn't something people typically shared with one another back then. My kids are eight years apart," Aunt Cindy said. "I had no problem getting pregnant with Andy, but it took about three and a half years with Leslie."

"I'm sorry to hear that you struggled. I never gave the age gap between your kids a second thought!"

A few days after we returned from Arizona, I went to see my new OB. The doctor flowed through the standard questions and did a wellness exam, and a nurse drew blood. I was disappointed to learn I would not have an ultrasound that day because the technician was not available. The OB told me to make a separate appointment for the ultrasound a week later.

A few days later, I got my complete blood count results back, a standard test that is done on every pregnant woman. My platelet level was slightly under the cutoff for normal, but my OB didn't feel it was a concern. I told her I would begin taking extra iron, because that seemed to help in the past. In the back of my mind, I wondered why my count would be low, despite delivering my son almost a year and a half ago. I decided to put it out of my mind and focus on enjoying the pregnancy instead. The cystic fibrosis blood test (a standard in California) result came back negative, which I assumed would be the case.

The day of my ultrasound appointment arrived. The technician was friendly and put me at ease. I had felt anxious in the week leading up to the appointment, but reminded myself that I was only thirty-five and had already had a successful pregnancy. The technician immediately found the fetal pole and yolk sac, and said I was eight weeks and two days pregnant. According to my last missed period, I should have been at ten weeks and three days, which at first caused a red flag. I then remembered that I had more than likely ovulated a few weeks late, so I could attribute it to that.

"What about the heartbeat?" I asked. "Does it seem normal?" My research told me that a heartbeat of 110 beats per minute or above was a positive thing.

"It's 175. It looks great! Everything else looks normal as well, although you have a fibroid on the outside of the uterus," she said.

"Yeah, I'm aware of that. It hasn't caused any problems so far, so I'm not concerned," I stated.

"Normally they don't when they're on the outside. They

can sometimes be painful during pregnancy though," she added.

"Yes, I remember hearing that. I was lucky that I never experienced anything during my first pregnancy." I thanked her for being so kind and forthcoming with information, and called Patrick.

"Well, everything looks great! I'm about eight weeks instead of ten, but I'm not surprised. I think I was correct in assuming I ovulated late, and that would explain the two-week discrepancy," I said.

"That's such a relief," my husband said. "I was waiting for your call and am glad everything turned out well."

"I have pictures I'll show you when you get home from work," I said.

"Sounds good. I look forward to seeing them."

I bought a special journal to keep a record of this pregnancy, just as I had done for Liam. I combed through the multiple options on Amazon, and decided on a fun and unique one called *The Belly Book* by Amy Krouse Rosenthal. When it arrived, I had fun filling in all the details I could remember up to that point, including the nausea, food cravings, ultrasound information, and general thoughts. The most exciting part was placing the ultrasound photos on the pages. I also wrote letters to the baby, as I had done for Liam. I shared details about when we found out I was pregnant, the anticipated due date, what activities our family had done over the past few months, and how excited I was to be a mom a second time.

At the eleven-week mark, I made up a fun way to tell my side of the family. I had fond memories of my dad singing "Here comes Peter Cottontail, hopping down the bunny trail…" each Easter when I was a kid. He enjoyed the holiday, and he gave us Easter baskets even when we were in high school, always signing, "Love, E. Bunny." My brother thought it was corny, but I found it endearing.

I wrote some lyrics, dressed Liam in a cute outfit, and had Patrick help him walk toward the video camera as I sang:

Here comes Liam Cottontail
Hopping Down the Bunny Trail
Excited to Tell You a Baby's on the Way

Liam was only seventeen months, so he got distracted and wandered off to the side, but we got the main point across. I uploaded it to You Tube, and made my sister-in-law promise to watch it with the whole family. I received a call soon afterward, congratulating us all, and wishing us the best.

The next task was when and how to tell Sandy and Pat the news. We planned to visit them Easter weekend, when I would be at twelve weeks. Easter is a very special time for my in-laws, so I thought this would be the ideal time to let them in on our little secret.

That weekend, my husband and I went shopping at the outlet malls, and I found a "Big Brother" shirt at one of the stores that I thought would be perfect to dress Liam in for the announcement. Easter morning we put on his shirt, sent him down the stairs, and waited for his grandparent's reaction. They didn't notice. We went outside for a mini Easter egg hunt, and they still didn't notice. We had to be blunt, and tell them to just look at Liam's shirt. They finally got it, and the expressions on their faces were priceless. They were over-joyed. This would be their third grandchild, and the second from my husband, who was their oldest.

11
DEVASTATION

*"You must give up the life you planned in order
to have the life that is waiting for you."*

\- Joseph Campbell

The following weekend, we flew to Denver to check on
the progress of our house project. I had also made a
thirteen-week genetic testing and ultrasound appointment at
the hospital where I delivered Liam. We knew we would be
living in Denver when the new baby was due, so we thought
it would be beneficial to have at least one appointment with
the facility.

On the last day of our visit, we went in for the ultrasound.
Eighteen-month-old Liam was zooming from one corner of
the genetic counselor's office to the other. We spent about
thirty minutes with the counselor. The only genetic concern

we had between both our families was that my husband had one cousin with Down syndrome. Although we understood this was not likely to be an issue, we agreed to do a simple blood test to find out.

Next, we were led into the room for the ultrasound. I could hardly wait to see the baby's progress since the last ultrasound at eight weeks. The technician flipped on the screen, and there was our baby. I smiled, and continued looking at it.

"Oh, it's not moving. Is it sleeping?" I asked.

"Just resting." The technician said. He looked around a bit longer, and then said he was going to bring in the doctor. When the doctor came in, she sat down next to me and placed her hand on my arm.

"I'm sorry," she said. "We couldn't find a heartbeat."

"No. No. Oh my God." I began to cry. I cried, and cried, and cried while my husband held my hand and asked the doctor, "Are you sure?"

I angrily turned my head toward him. "YES, she's SURE!" I cried and cried some more as Liam busied himself with a toy on the floor.

She stated in a soft voice, "You should be thirteen weeks, and it looks like growth ceased right around twelve weeks. I can't find anything that would give me an answer as to why this happened, but I can tell you that in about 50 percent of these cases, the reason is a chromosomal abnormality."

After spending some more time with us discussing a D&C procedure, she excused herself and allowed us to spend some time alone.

"I can't believe this is happening," I said to my husband through my tears. "I just can't believe this. Oh my God. Why did this happen? We were just about out of the first trimester!"

We were both distraught but knew we had to move out of the room, and more importantly, attend to the child we already had. I was in a fog on the car ride home. I stared out the window and silently attempted to accept what had just happened.

I switched in to operational mode because I felt like I was emotionally losing control. I needed to make a decision about where and when to have the D&C done. We were flying back to California the following day, and I didn't know what kind of care was available there.

When we got back to the house, I spent the next few hours calling various facilities that could perform a D&C. The most obvious choice was the hospital we had just visited. I could go in the next day, but that would mean I would have to stay in Denver alone, going through the procedure without Patrick, who needed to fly back to California for work. Also, what would we do with Liam during that time? Neither one of us had family in the area, so we would need to make arrangements for him. My head was spinning, and I didn't know what to do. However, the deal was sealed when I was informed that the cost of the procedure would be $2,500. At this point, my grief turned to anger.

"I refuse to pay $2,500 to walk away with nothing! I've already had a baby taken from me. I understand this has to be done, but not at *that* cost! We need to look elsewhere," I said.

Patrick assured me he would stay with me in Denver if we decided to do the procedure there. I continued to call other places, both in Denver and in California. I finally settled on a Planned Parenthood location about a thirty-minute drive from where we were living in California, and I made an appointment for that Saturday morning. We could all fly back to California as scheduled the next day, my husband could return to work on time, and my in-laws could watch Liam.

I called one of my dearest friends, Sarah, to tell her the devastating news. She immediately left work to be by my side, and embraced me on the front steps of our house. She didn't say anything; she just held me while I unleashed even more tears.

I appreciated that she didn't say anything like, "It's going to be okay. At least you have one." The only thing I remember her saying is, "I'm so, so sorry, Jen." In that very moment, I believe she understood that silence was what I needed most, even though she didn't have any children of her own, and had not experienced a miscarriage. She is a wise soul.

I then called my dad to tell him the news. My dad had been the family "go to" person for a lot of my educational, career, and financial concerns, but never for emotional support. I had grown up without hugs or hearing, "I love you," and we never discussed our feelings. In the past, conversations with my dad had involved the weather, politics, health concerns, or my son. It never got too deep. That day, he listened patiently as I told my story. My mom never played any type of support roll, and I did not expect it would be any different that day.

We still had to meet with the general contractor who came to the house to discuss the work that had been completed while we were gone, and the plans for the upcoming months. I did my part, walking through the house and saying, "This looks great. Can we change this? Can we add to that?" I tried to cover up my broken heart and anguish over the news we had received only a few hours prior. I smiled and asked her to take a picture of our three-person family in front of the house.

Our final visitor of the trip was a friend who was getting married in a month. He excitedly described the wedding location and honeymoon plans, and we responded as enthusiastically as we could. I recall sitting at our dining room table thinking, "*There's a dead baby in me right now.*" I felt a gripping emotional pain as I smiled and wished our friend the best with his wedding.

12

GRIEF AND ANGER

*"The enemy always fights you the hardest when he knows
God has something great in your future."*

- Pastor Joel Osteen

On the plane ride back to California, I sat in the window seat staring at the clouds, and I struggled to grasp the reality of what was happening. I wanted to wake up from this dark nightmare. I wanted to believe there was still a life growing inside me. I wanted to scream, and I wanted to run away. I wanted to bury my head in a pillow and sleep for a very long time. I wanted my baby's heart to start beating again. My thoughts raced.

"How could this have happened? We had a perfectly normal ultrasound at eight weeks. I understand miscarriages happen in the first trimester, but my baby had grown to twelve weeks gestation. What went wrong?" I couldn't help but wonder if I had somehow inadvertently caused the miscarriage. I recalled the day Liam and I had taken a long, brisk walk to Target, and wondered if I had gotten my heart rate up too high. I scrutinized what I had eaten over the weeks, and wondered if the turkey sandwich had caused a Listeria infection. I wondered if I had worked out too hard at the gym. I blamed myself.

As we walked to baggage claim at the Ontario International Airport in California, I thought about the play date I had scheduled with my friend from the mom's club that afternoon. I mustered up the courage to call her, and broke down while telling her the news. She said she understood if I didn't want to come over, but encouraged me to do whatever I needed to. I decided that being around a friend would be comforting.

When we walked into our apartment, one of the first things I noticed was the congratulations card that we had received from my mother-in-law the previous week, stating how excited she was about the pregnancy, and wishing us the best. I ripped the card from the shelf and threw it in the recycle bin. I then went straight to our bedroom to retrieve the Belly Book I had so lovingly filled out, and threw it in the garbage. I deleted Liam's video announcement. I felt out of control…again.

The Mom's Club was the only support system I had in California. I soon received a phone call from the club president.

"Jen, I just wanted to say how sorry I am to hear about your loss. I know this might not be what you need to hear right now, but I also had a miscarriage between my first and second children. I had a D&C, which is what I'm assuming you'll be having."

"You did?" I asked. "You're the first person I've talked to who can relate. I'm really concerned about it. I don't know what to expect."

Dilation and curettage (D&C) involves the widening/opening of the cervix and surgical removal of part of the lining of the uterus and/or contents of the uterus by scraping and scooping. Because she was a nurse, and had gone through this procedure herself, she was able to describe to me what I could expect. I felt relieved. My friend offered to support me in any way she could, and I was grateful. She also reported that she successfully conceived about two months after her D&C, and she knew many others who had as well. I spoke with another group member who said she too had conceived within a few months after her miscarriage. I was told that your body "wants to be pregnant again," so a large number of women are successful soon afterwards. I hoped I would experience the same.

One of the most painful calls was to my mother-in-law. Patrick and I sat on our bed, and he revealed the news. Without being on the listening end, I could sense that her heart was breaking for the grandchild she would never meet, and for the anguish that her son and daughter-in-law must be experiencing.

A few days later, a sympathy fruit basket arrived from my brother's family. It was a heartfelt gesture, and one that had been carefully thought out. My sister-in-law knew how much I tried to lead a healthy lifestyle, so I was certain that a lot of care had gone into selecting the gift. My heart lifted slightly. It helped knowing we were being thought about and cared for.

Sympathy cards and emails flowed in, and the two that had the greatest impact on me were the cards from extended family members who disclosed they had been through miscarriages as well. One had occurred at least thirty-five years prior, and the other in the past two years. I was so grateful to them for sharing with me. It allowed me to feel that I wasn't the only one. I was later astounded to learn that out of twenty-five members of our mom's club, seven of us had a miscarriage—more than 25 percent of the group.

I didn't know anything about miscarriage at the time. I thought it was something that happened to other people. I thought it was something that happened in the first five to eight weeks of pregnancy. I didn't know how to "properly" grieve. I didn't know how to hide the grief from Liam. I just knew how to lie on my bed and cry, and cry, and cry for the baby I would never meet. I thought, *What would he or she have looked like? Was it a boy or a girl? How would he or she have interacted with Liam?* I knew how to be angry and engrossed with the fact that we had been through what I considered a lot to have Liam, and now this!

The grief and anger became overwhelming. I had to do something to help ease the sting. I drove out to the beach in Santa Monica, knowing the ocean always has a calming effect on me. I walked to the cliffs overlooking the Pacific Ocean and Pacific Coast Highway, and released my baby's soul. I told him or her that we would meet some day. It was all I knew to do, and it felt like enough. I walked down to the beach, allowing the warm, soft sand to cover my bare feet. The April weather allowed me to comfortably sit on a blanket, and listen to the waves rolling in and out. I meditated on peace and comfort, while feeling the sun on my face, and listening to the sounds of the birds above.

I returned my mother-in-law's phone message from earlier in the day.

"I just can't stop crying," I said gulping for air.

"Neither can I," she said.

I've always known my mother-in-law to be a positive, loving, kind, and strong person. As much as this tragedy had rocked my world, it was obvious it had rocked hers as well. It was the first time I'd heard her cry.

"I'm just so sorry this happened, Jen, and I've been praying for you. I know your little baby is in Heaven with the angels."

"Thank you. I appreciate that, and thank you for agreeing to keep Liam overnight, so we can go to our appointment." Sandy was the closest person to a mother figure in my life at the time. I was grateful to have her love and support.

13

PUSHING THROUGH

"The greatest glory in living lies not in never falling,
but in rising every time we fall."

- Nelson Mandela

Planned Parenthood said to arrive at 6:30 a.m. on Saturday, April 21, 2012. Liam was safely sleeping at my in-laws, so it was just Patrick and me. When we arrived, it was still dark. We walked up to the front door, where about three couples were already in line. They were not invited inside, because there was not enough space to accommodate everyone in the waiting area. I was told there was a receptionist taking information, who would then buzz each person into the facility through a security door. This meant that the three couples, along with the growing line of arrivals behind us, all were forced to wait outside. It is not cold in California at the end of April, so I was not physically uncomfortable. As for the emotional side of things, the crying had started to decrease. I felt I had made peace on that cliff overlooking the ocean, and was ready to move forward. I felt as strong as I was able to in that given moment.

We waited outside for about fifteen minutes before I noticed the protesters on the other side of the sidewalk, holding signs stating:

It's not too late.

Choose life. Your mother did.

Abortion is a painful choice.

It was the first time I realized that the majority of the people standing in line were there for an abortion. They weren't removing babies without a heartbeat. They were ending unwanted pregnancies with strong heartbeats.

My husband became increasingly agitated and angry at the protestors.

"They don't have a right to be here," he grunted under his breath.

"I think they do," I said. "They're not on public property, and they, unfortunately, have a right to their opinion."

"Don't they know that we're not here to kill our baby? Don't they know that we didn't choose for this to happen to us? I'm going to go over and say something."

"No, we need to leave it alone," I said. "We know what we're here for. It doesn't matter what anyone else thinks. This is hard enough, and confronting them will only make it harder."

"You're right," he agreed. "I just wish they would let us wait inside so we wouldn't have to see them."

Once inside, I filled out the required forms, checking the box that called for general anesthesia. I opted to be completely sedated during this experience, so I would have no memory of it. For reasons that were never clearly explained to us, my husband was not allowed to be with me at any stage of the process, which could last for up to six hours.

I was finally called back, instructed to lock all my belongings in a locker, and was led to an ultrasound room. The technician confirmed that the fetus was at twelve weeks gestation, and that it did not have a heartbeat. This is when I realized that all the other ultrasounds the technician performed that morning were for fetuses that were still alive, and I was shocked.

"Wow," I said. "How do you deal with seeing all these fetuses, knowing they won't be alive in a few hours?" I tried as hard as I could to phrase the question nonjudgmentally, as it was certainly not my intention to judge her job. In fact, I empathized with her.

"You know, you just get used to it," she said. "That doesn't mean it's always easy, though. I just try to put myself in the girl's shoes and realize it's her choice to make."

I was then led to an examination room where I was handed what I believe was Cytotec to dilate my cervix. I had done a lot of research about Cytotec before my son's birth and was not overly thrilled about taking the medication. However, the nurse assured me it was absolutely safe and is frequently used for D&Cs, and she said the staff would keep a watchful eye on me. I was sent to a waiting room while the drug took effect. There was a TV, a few magazines, and about five women who I guessed to be between the ages of eighteen and thirty sitting in chairs. None of us spoke to one another. None of us read any of the magazines. Most stared blankly at the TV. I can only imagine what they must have been thinking, and I can honestly say that I wasn't judging any of them. I did not condone what they were doing, but I reminded myself that I was not privy to the details of their situations, and it was none of my business.

I was led to the operating room where I met the doctor and nurses who would perform the D&C. The doctor said how sorry he was about my situation, which I appreciated. One of the nurses assured me that this particular doctor was one of their best, and that I was in very capable hands. She then told me they were going to administer Propofol for the general anesthesia.

"Like the drug Michael Jackson's doctor used?" I asked, trying to make light of an extremely challenging situation.

"Yes," the nurse explained. "It's the same one, and completely safe."

The next thing I remember was waking up in the recovery room. One of the nurses brought me crackers and a Ginger Ale.

The girl in the bed next to mine was sobbing as she awoke and became aware of her surroundings. "I don't want to do it. Can I take it back?" she cried.

My heart broke for her, despite my deep desire to have been in her position of having a baby with a beating heart. I assumed her decision hadn't been an easy one and her road to emotional recovery likely would be treacherous.

A nurse gave me a standard Rho(D) immune globulin injection, due to my Rh negative blood type. It was a precaution against a situation called Rh incompatibility, which could affect future pregnancies and cause hemolytic disease in a newborn. I got my recovery instructions and went on my way. My husband and I drove to my in-laws where we were reunited with Liam who was unaware that anything had happened.

14
MOVING FORWARD

"Faith is taking the first step even when you
don't see the whole staircase."

- Martin Luther King, Jr.

I decided to visit my family in Chicago. I still felt lonely and isolated living in California, and I wanted some family support. When I arrived, no one said a word about my miscarriage. It was as if it never happened, and I felt maybe everyone thought I had gotten over it and moved forward. My dad and mom did not acknowledge that I was grieving. As upsetting as this was, I realized those who have not experienced such a loss cannot begin to comprehend what it feels like.

I remembered the time when my then thirty-four-year-old girlfriend informed me of her diagnosis of breast cancer.

I was shocked and felt horrible for her, but I didn't know how to be there for her or what to say. I think I sent her a magazine article on nutrition after chemotherapy or something to that effect. I can only imagine how unhelpful it was. I also recalled a friend who mentioned that his sister had twins, and one of the babies had died in the neonatal intensive care unit at five months old. I responded, "How horrible! I can't imagine experiencing something like that. I feel so awful for your sister!" Although this was an appropriate response, I wasn't able to grasp the emotional impact. I am grateful my miscarriage allowed me to deepen my sense of empathy.

One night, we all sat at the dinner table discussing nothing of importance when my mom muttered a negative comment under her breath about something my dad had said, a common occurrence throughout the years. All the emotional build-up from the past few weeks came to a head at that moment, and I lost it when my mom left the room.

I turned to my dad and said, "I can't believe I just lost a baby, and she hasn't even acknowledged it! Is she not able to comprehend it? Does she even KNOW, or does her dementia get in the way?"

My dad confirmed that she knew, but he added nothing else.

I realized how strongly I was grieving, and how past issues with my mom still had the ability to affect my emotional well-being. I would have given anything to have an understanding, loving, supportive mom to hold my hand through this awful journey, to tell me everything was going to be okay, that I would survive this and grow stronger for it. Even if she had been able to say she was there for me if I needed her, or she was sorry to hear what I was going through, it would have helped. I know sometimes it's better to say nothing, but this was my MOM, and I expected more from her. I still had work to do on letting go and forgiving.

Seven weeks after the D&C, while we were visiting Patrick's friend, my period started. His friend's wife was in her early forties, and had experienced an early miscarriage before she had her baby. She described the experience as "not a big deal," saying it was her partner who had had difficulty with it. She said she knew she would get pregnant soon after, and she did—two months after. I became hopeful that I knew yet another person who got pregnant so soon after a miscarriage.

As hopeful as I was, I became triggered by comments I considered insensitive. In the months after the miscarriage, I heard a slew of supposed "comforting" comments, each of which singed my already fried emotions:

At least you have one.

At least you know you can get pregnant.

It was probably meant to be.

It will get better.

As grateful as I was to have at least one child, I was grieving for the one I had recently lost, and my delightful son, unfortunately, could not take away that pain. I knew I could get pregnant, but was now aware that I wasn't able to remain pregnant for some unknown reason. This was not very reassuring. "It was probably meant to be," seemed to state that the baby more than likely had a chromosomal abnormality, and the miscarriage was a way of taking care of it. I didn't know that for certain, and neither did the person who said it. My rational mind knew things would get better, but I felt patronized being told so. Although I knew people just didn't know what to say, I wished they could instead say they were thinking about me, or that I seemed to be doing a great job of handling the situation.

Approximately a month after my period returned, we moved back to Denver for good. My friend, Sarah, who was so supportive during my miscarriage, flew out to California to drive back with us to help with twenty-month-old Liam. We stopped for a lunch break in the interesting casino town of Laughlin, Nevada, where it was a balmy 100 degrees Fahrenheit, then drove to Williamsburg, Arizona to rest for the night.

The next day, we visited the Grand Canyon, a breathtaking sight. We then traveled to Lake Powell and stayed one night, and then drove on to Durango, Colorado to visit and stay with Patrick's former boss at his beautiful home in the woods. Finally, we explored Taos, New Mexico and arrived in Denver just a few weeks after the July 2012 wildfires. We could see the haze in the air, and although we felt for the people who had been affected, we were grateful our friends and extended family were safe.

I began keeping track of my cycles again, and was pleasantly surprised when my cycle lasted only thirty-two days, putting me in the normal range. Although I wasn't pregnant yet, I did wonder if my body was regulating itself, and hoped we might have a chance at getting pregnant naturally. Despite feeling hopeful, I still made an appointment with my reproductive endocrinologist to discuss a plan.

Patrick did not attend the consultation. He was still traveling back and forth to California. Since he was out of town four days of every week, the chance of correctly timing ovulation with intercourse would be a challenge, especially with my longer, unpredictable cycles. However, I was willing to take the chance that we might time it correctly before moving ahead with medication or treatments. When I described the miscarriage to my RE, she looked up from what she was reading with wide eyes.

"It happened at twelve weeks? That seems a little late in the first trimester."

"I know," I replied. "That's what I thought as well."

"Did they test the tissue?" she asked.

"No. I heard it could cost $500 to $1,000, and that if it was a girl, the test might come back inconclusive or normal."

During my research, I discovered the tissue that is tested often can be that of the mother, so the test is pointless. Also, since this was my first miscarriage, I did not feel testing was crucial.

"I'm going to recommend a fasting glucose blood test, as well as an insulin blood test to determine if we might be looking at an issue that can cause recurrent miscarriages," my doctor said.

"Sounds good to me. I don't want the same thing to happen when I become pregnant again."

"I'd also like to test your FSH and estradiol levels on day three of your cycle," she said.

The glucose and insulin blood tests came back in the normal range. My follicle stimulating hormone (FSH) level came back at 5.5, my lowest result ever, putting me in the "excellent" category. The lower the number, the higher the chance of becoming pregnant. My estradiol level fell just short of the lower-end cutoff, but my RE did not feel it was relevant enough to discuss with me.

We agreed I would try the lowest dose of the ovulation-inducing medication letrozole again. However, we agreed that I would not come in for ultrasound monitoring. Instead, we would time ovulation on our own to save money. Unfortunately, my home ovulation predictor kit indicated I had not ovulated that month, and to make matters even worse, I had a thirty-nine day cycle, putting me once again in the abnormal range.

I had joined a mom's group in my neighborhood when we got back to Denver, and was invited to a mom's night out at a local restaurant, where I met Lindsay. We had a lot in common. Lindsay was not only a psychological counselor, but also someone who had been struggling with infertility. She had a colorful story to share regarding her successful in vitro fertilization at the Colorado Center for Reproductive Medicine, resulting in her daughter, who was slightly younger than Liam. We began meeting for coffee and play dates, and established a friendship and a close bond.

No one else I knew was struggling with infertility, so I didn't have anyone who could relate. I bonded with Lindsay over shared struggles with being stay-at-home moms, trying to successfully raise toddlers while experiencing the emotional roller coaster of infertility, trying to keep our marriages and friendships intact through it all, and our efforts to have a second child. I appreciated so very much that Lindsay could relate to my personal struggle.

For the next three months, Patrick and I tried letrozole medication and timed intercourse, with no luck. I even took a desperate road trip out to California with the intention of being with Patrick during what we thought would be ovulation time. Each time my period arrived, I would sink into despair for a few days, then pick myself up and move forward.

I turned thirty-six, yet another year older, and was reminded that the baby I miscarried would have been born shortly before my birthday. I was saddened by the fact that we were no closer to having that baby in our arms, but hopeful things would turn out for the best. A mutual friend delivered her baby approximately the same day that I would have delivered mine, and it was painful to see the newborn pictures posted on Facebook.

I received notice by mail that my RE had left the practice. I had the choice of staying with this practice, or moving on. As this was the practice that helped me achieve a successful pregnancy the first time around, and it was one of the most affordable practices, I decided to stay with it. However, I would be forced to work with the doctor I didn't like—the one who told me to stop exercising and eat ice cream. I had researched the average number of cycles it should take to get pregnant with oral medication only, and was aware that I was exhausting this option. I assumed the new doctor and I would discuss intrauterine inseminations (IUIs) at our consultation.

According to a pamphlet I picked up at the RE office, the objective of an IUI is to put sperm directly into the uterus to facilitate fertilization of an egg. Those who are ovulating normally, have open fallopian tubes, and have a normal uterine cavity are the most successful. The goal is to stimulate the release of, at most, two eggs. IUIs are known to be most successful in couples with no obvious cause of infertility, and the success rates are between 10 to 20 percent per cycle. Doctors often recommend two to three cycles of IUI, and if these are not successful, IVF is suggested.

I came to our consultation prepared with a list of questions for the new RE.

"Why haven't I become pregnant after three rounds of oral medication if I'm ovulating, my fallopian tubes are open, and my husband has a normal sperm count?" I asked.

"Well ... age," she stated.

"Age? But I'm only thirty-six, and I have a great FSH level," I said.

"As you probably know, fertility begins to decline in the thirties, and especially in the mid-thirties," she explained.

What about all those people who become pregnant in their late thirties and early forties? I wondered, but I didn't ask. This RE's personality was more abrupt than my previous one, and I got the sense she didn't want to explain further.

"Is my actual diagnosis PCOS? I assumed I fit into the unexplained category."

"Technically you don't meet the definition of polycystic ovarian syndrome, but it is quite possible that you have polycystic ovaries, making it more difficult to ovulate."

"Shouldn't the medication help with that? Every time I take medication, I ovulate. I just don't seem to get pregnant."

"Sometimes we need a more aggressive approach, such as IUIs," she explained.

"Would I have to do the IUI with fresh sperm, or could we use frozen?" I asked. "My husband is out of town four full days each week, and I can't guarantee he'll be in town at the right time."

"Frozen sperm can be used, but it has a slightly lower success rate," she said.

"Would I use oral medication or injectable medication?" I asked. "What is the difference in success rates?"

"Injectable medication results in slightly higher success rates, but it is more expensive. Whereas a medication only cycle can be $700 to $800, an injectable medication cycle can be $2,000 to $3,000."

"Since we are paying out of pocket for everything, I'd like to attempt at least three IUIs with just oral medication, and I would like to start as soon as possible," I said.

"Okay. Your husband will need to provide a sperm sample to be frozen for future use if needed."

Patrick provided the sample the week my in-laws, who were unaware of anything we were going through, flew into town for Thanksgiving. Although he was forty-four at the time, his "semen cryopreservation report" was comparable to someone in his twenties or thirties. In fact, the sample was so robust and abundant that the laboratory was able to split it in half, leaving us with an extra sample for the future.

As excited as I was to move forward, I struggled with the news that more and more people I knew were becoming pregnant. Patrick's friend's wife, whom we had visited only four months prior (and who, by this time, had a six month old), announced on Facebook that she was pregnant and expecting a boy. I sent a congratulatory email, crying as I hit send. I was done with Facebook. It had become painful over the months to see all the ultrasound photos, belly bumps, newborn pictures, and babies that were being born around the same time that I would have delivered mine. Unfortunately, I cut off social contact with a lot of people, but fortunately, it allowed some of my anxiety and grief to subside.

15

TRIALS AND TRIBULATIONS

"Never surrender in the face of challenges. Challenges are just the Universe's way of making sure you earn, and deserve, the success you are striving for. If you work vigorously with persistence and dedication while connecting to the force that surrounds you, destiny will provide you with the attainment of your desire."

- Richard A. Singer

As I prepared for the IUI, I became concerned about the number of follicles I might produce, but was reassured that I would be monitored via ultrasound. I ended up producing only one large follicle. I injected myself with Ovidrel to trigger ovulation, and arrived at the office for the procedure. Patrick was in town, and was able to provide a fresh sperm sample. The "sperm wash report" indicated there were 54,900,000 sperm (with 10,000,000 the minimum for the best success rate), so we felt confident! I uncovered plenty of first-time success stories during my hours of Google research.

Of course, there also were many stories of second and third time successes, so I was convinced we would be successful within at least three attempts. My husband's sperm were strong, I had previously birthed a healthy baby, and there was nothing medically wrong with me that would prevent me from becoming pregnant. The doctor said to take a pregnancy test in fourteen days.

I didn't need to wait that long, because my period arrived nine days after the procedure. I was crushed. That left us with only two more times before we would need to discuss moving on to IVF.

I decided it was time to seek additional support, as my emotional well-being was starting to unravel. This is when I found an online support community through RESOLVE, "the National Infertility Association" at www.resolve.org. The RESOLVE site listed a number of local, in-person support groups. However, I was not able to attend any due to Patrick's out-of-town work schedule, and I understood that it would not be appropriate to bring Liam. The next best scenario was the online chat boards. I set up my profile and chose which specific groups to join from the wealth of subgroups:

- Newly diagnosed
- IUI / IVF and high-tech procedures
- High FSH
- Secondary infertility
- Infertility at 40+

- IVF veterans
- Third party reproduction
- Adoption
- Living childfree
- Taking a break
- Research
- Male perspective
- Pregnancy loss
- Financial issues
- Insurance issues
- Seeking treatment outside the U.S.
- Friends and family
- What's happening at RESOLVE
- Walk of Hope
- Media alerts
- Advocacy
- Volunteers

I was astounded at how many groups were offered, and overwhelmed with which ones to choose. I also was impressed that an organization was willing to put forth the effort to assist those of us struggling with infertility. We were in the middle of attempting IUIs, so I decided to join the "IUI / IVF and high-tech procedure" group. This group appeared to have the highest membership and largest number of posts, so I assumed I would gain great feedback. I wondered if I technically fit into the secondary infertility category, and did a bit more research. According to RESOLVE'S definition of secondary infertility, I did not. It is defined as "the inability to become pregnant, or to carry a pregnancy to term, following the birth of one or more biological children. The birth of the first child does not involve any assisted reproductive technologies or fertility medications." Liam WAS conceived with fertility medications, so I actually fit into the primary infertility category, which seemed strange. It didn't matter. I stayed with the IUI group.

I spent a lot of time reading posts, and sometimes I would reply to them, but mostly I perused. Maybe I didn't feel I belonged on this type of site, or maybe I needed to get a better feel for the group first, or maybe I didn't want to commit. I didn't believe I'd be involved with the group for very long.

I didn't have much time to think about or reply to many posts, as we planned to fly to California to spend the 2012 Christmas holiday with Patrick's family. None of the family was aware of what we were going through, because we chose to keep it to ourselves. However, it was obvious I was behaving differently. I found it difficult to take pleasure in the types of activities I had in the past, such as spending time at the beach and having down time with the family. I secretly cried a lot during that vacation, but hid my tears and my medication from the others. I bet they suspected something was going on as I struggled to smile and participate in conversation. Infertility can be an all-consuming challenge.

2013

Fortunately, we planned a short road trip for the beginning of the New Year 2013 up the central coast. We visited the Santa Barbara Zoo, and I recall feeling blessed that we had the ability to take Liam there, as opposed to not having a child. I was always well-aware of the fact that I was fortunate to have him, but it was now going on fifteen months since we started trying to have a second, and eight months since the miscarriage.

We spent a few days in Pismo Beach, taking side trips for hiking in San Luis Obispo, and then on to Avila Beach. On the way back, we stopped at the Monarch Butterfly Grove, just south of Pismo Beach. There were thousands of Monarch butterflies, mostly sunning themselves in the trees. We borrowed a pair of the ranger's binoculars to take a closer look at these majestic yellow and black creatures. Not long after we arrived, a butterfly landed on my arm. I was shocked, and asked the ranger how often this occurs. She explained that it's not a common occurrence. I gave my husband a knowing look.

"This has to mean something. This must be a sign that we're going to get pregnant this year. I just know it," I said. "You heard her. She said butterflies hardly ever land on people, and this one chose to land on me. Take a picture!"

The date was January 3, 2013. I made a mental note not to forget.

Shortly after we returned to Denver, we geared up for a second IUI. Although I had taken 7.5 milligrams daily of letrozole to stimulate ovulation—about three times the normal dose—I produced only one large follicle. This was not necessarily a negative, but more follicles produce more eggs, and raise the odds of becoming pregnant.

Once or twice a week, I went to Denver Community Acupuncture for treatments. I met one on one with a practitioner for the first appointment to discuss my personal concerns, but after that, I received treatments in the community room among four or five other patients. This was an affordable way to get in a few treatments per week. My acupuncturist, too, was struggling to get pregnant. I found her to be knowledgeable about my course of treatment and empathetic to my concerns.

My acupuncturist soon referred me to her friend, Brooke, who had successfully conceived both of her children via first-time IVF attempts with CCRM. Although I had decided not to use CCRM when I was trying to get pregnant with my first, this time I was feeling open to the possibility. When I met up with Brooke, she was adamant that I switch facilities.

I had watched multiple episodes of the reality show "Giuliana and Bill," but was not aware that this also was the facility they used for their attempt at pregnancy. By this time, I knew they had successfully conceived via a gestational carrier and had a baby at home. If celebrities had chosen to work with this facility, I figured it must have a good reputation. When I called to book my consultation, there were no openings for weeks. I hoped I would be forced to cancel that appointment because we would become pregnant.

For our second IUI attempt, my husband's travel schedule dictated that he would be out of town on procedure day, so we used his frozen sperm sample. The thaw process went smoothly, but this time the sample had just under half the total number of sperm that we had used for our first IUI. The nurse reassured me that the sample contained twice the amount necessary for a successful outcome, but it was obvious that a fresh sample was optimal. The nurse was kind and genuine throughout everything, and her empathetic nature allowed me to relax and have hope. She reminded me that a large number of people successfully get pregnant after three to four IUIs, and I felt reassured.

Before leaving the office, the nurse instructed me to take oral progesterone for the next few days to alleviate my luteal phase defect concerns. I don't believe the reproductive facility staff agreed with my concern, but my RE was more than willing to prescribe the medication. The idea of progesterone support resulting in successful pregnancies is controversial. Some schools of thought believe the support can save a pregnancy that otherwise would result in a miscarriage, and others believe it has no effect whatsoever. I figured it couldn't hurt.

The plan was to continue taking the progesterone and take a home pregnancy test in two weeks. If it was negative, I would stop taking the progesterone and my period would arrive. Before I had a chance to take the test, my period arrived with a vengeance at a friend's Super Bowl party. I remember noticing pre-menstrual symptoms but tried to focus on the party and chat with people while periodically excusing myself to go to the bathroom to see if it had arrived. Not only did it come, but it was accompanied by uncomfortable cramps beyond the norm. I blamed the cramps on the progesterone, and began planning our next efforts. We had just completed our second failed IUI. According to my "timeline," we had only one more to go before a different course of action would become necessary.

In February 2013, a year after we thought we were on our way to having our second child, and almost a year after my miscarriage, I was hit hard with the realization that I was not in control. Up to the point when I first tried to get pregnant, I had moved my life in the direction I chose, even if that meant going a different direction than I originally thought. Never had I encountered such an obstacle to something I so desperately wanted. I became isolated and backed off from socializing with friends. I was in a rut, and didn't want to expose anyone to my negative thoughts. Raising a toddler during this time was exceptionally challenging, and I often wondered how Liam would be affected by my bouts of anxiety and depression.

I sought out, and began meeting with, a psychotherapist who specialized in "reproductive mental wellness" issues, including infertility, pregnancy loss, and pregnancy after loss. I carefully researched and chose this counselor due to her specialties. Although I got the feeling she had not experienced infertility herself, she was able to meet me where I was at and empathized with my situation. However, it made me all the more determined to become an "infertility expert" so I would be able to relate fully to what my future clients were experiencing. I believe these multiple therapy sessions were necessary to my emotional well-being, and I was thankful I had been humble enough to realize it. My therapist and I worked to get to a place where I could accept my situation, and look forward to the future with hope and faith.

As Liam got older, people began asking if I was working, or whether I was thinking about starting up my psychotherapy private practice again. I struggled to answer these questions as honestly as possible, without revealing our infertility challenges to those who were unaware. I assumed I would get pregnant soon, so I continued to put off working. I didn't feel I had the time or the emotional resources to rebuild my private practice while trying to get pregnant. I wasn't in the right frame of mind to do it. I put off people's questions with a vague, "I'd like to start my practice up some day in the future, but I'm not sure when."

I kept up my state-required continuing education so I could keep my license and attended trainings and networking meetings to earn some credits. At one networking meeting, the facilitator created time for introductions and sharing. As I listened to one introduction after another, the specialties began to blend together: "anxiety, depression, substance abuse..."

My ears perked up when I heard one of the participants say, "Infertility, pregnancy, and baby loss." As the meeting concluded, I made a point of introducing myself to this colleague, and asked for her contact information. She handed me her business card with a warm smile, and encouraged me to be in touch.

Christina was the second friend I made who was able to relate to what I was experiencing. We met at a coffee shop, and through tears, shared our infertility stories. Christina happened to be working with CCRM, the facility I had an appointment with the following month. She explained that she and her husband had tried for the past ten years to have a baby. Their first IVF attempt at a Texas reproductive facility resulted in a miscarriage at eight weeks, and the second attempt resulted in a baby girl who died upon delivery at twenty-four weeks gestation.

As I listened to her story, my heart broke into a million pieces. I was unable to comprehend how someone could endure so much and appear so strong, at least on the outside. We continued to meet on a regular basis, and established a mutually supportive friendship.

My thoughts about our third and final IUI attempt in February 2013 were varied. On one hand, I felt defeated, having already experienced two failed IUIs, and was realistic about the possibility of a third failure. As with the first and second IUI attempts, I wasn't willing to pay for injectable medication. It was a lot more expensive, and the odds of an actual conception were not much higher. I knew if the third IUI failed, our appointment with CCRM was only two weeks away, and I would get the insight of experts there.

Fortunately, we had another back-up frozen sperm sample, because we needed it. Patrick would once again be in California the day of the procedure. I was hopeful, mostly because I was aware that a large number of people are successful by their third or fourth attempt.

Before I was due to take a pregnancy test, and despite having taken progesterone, I started bleeding again. I was angry. *"Why does this keep happening? I thought we had a good chance during each and every attempt! Did the facility time the IUI correctly?"*

I was so distraught that our final attempt had failed, but was looking forward to meeting up with a girlfriend that night for dinner and drinks. She listened intently as I described our fruitless attempts at conception over the past several months. It felt good to vent, and I left with high anticipation of the consultation with CCRM.

16

WORLD CLASS FACILITY

"To learn to trust you must experiment being neutral about what happens in your life. You don't have to see things in a positive light. Just stop seeing them in a negative light. Stop imposing your expectations on the events and circumstances of your life. Just let life unfold and see what happens."

                                  - Paul Ferrini

While waiting for our initial consultation appointment with CCRM, I researched the facility more thoroughly. I discovered that not only had it existed for twenty-four years, but its success rates were among the highest in the world. The main location was only a twenty-minute drive from my house, and it offered comprehensive chromosomal screening (CCS).

A few days into my period after our third IUI failure, and a few days before the initial consultation appointment with CCRM, my period was a lot heavier than normal. I noticed strong cramping, and small clots that I attributed to the progesterone I had taken. Still, my symptoms were definitely out of the norm compared to previous cycles.

Patrick was working in California during the appointment. I didn't see this as too much of an obstacle, because I was the one who had spent hours of time researching infertility and assisted reproductive technologies. I would pass on what I learned to my husband, and he would provide feedback. However, I became concerned about bringing my then two-and-a-half-year-old son into the waiting room with other patients. I recognized how challenging infertility could be when you don't have a child, and I didn't want to upset anyone. I also became concerned about having a serious conversation with my doctor without interruption.

I took many steps to prepare for this initial consultation. I knew we would be spending a lot of money to work with CCRM, and I wanted to be as thorough as possible. I requested my medical records from all the facilities that had been involved in our infertility journey: the reproductive endocrinologist office in Denver, the reproductive endocrinologist office in California, the OB/GYN office in California where my prenatal care was done, the hospital where my miscarriage was discovered, and Planned Parenthood where my D&C took place. I ensured that all these facilities sent records to CCRM, and that CCRM received them. I also prepared a list of questions for my CCRM doctor. I had done so much research that I felt like a mini-expert in the field!

I knew well in advance which of the five doctors I would be working with, as I had hand picked him myself. His bio was impressive and was the reason I chose to work with him. According to the CCRM website, www.colocrm.com, Dr.

Surrey was a board-certified reproductive endocrinologist who had a lot of impressive credits in his experience, including being named one of America's Top Doctors for Women by Women's Health Magazine.

The facility was located in a two-story, stand-alone building, with its own parking lot, and a beautiful view of the Rocky Mountains. Upon entering the building, I couldn't help but notice a calming waterfall sign with the facility's name on it. There were two reception desks and two waiting areas, one to the left and one to the right. Dr. Surrey greeted me warmly, and his demeanor quickly put me at ease. He greeted Liam as well, and appeared comfortable about letting him play on the floor. We began discussing my reproductive history.

"You took 10 milligrams of letrozole for your last IUI?" he asked.

"Um … yes," I sheepishly admitted. "I produced only one follicle until I started taking 10 milligrams, when I produced two."

"I would not have put you on that high of a dosage," he said. He then acknowledged my list of questions, and answered them one by one.

"Is it possible that scarring from the D&C after my miscarriage almost a year ago might be preventing pregnancy?" I asked. "And what about the possibility of blocked fallopian tubes? I had an HSG two-and-a-half years ago that was normal though."

"Both of those are a possibility. One of our standard work-up tests is an HSG. This should tell us if there is any scarring or any tube blockage," he said.

"I have a fibroid on the outside of my uterus. Is there any chance it would be preventing pregnancy?" I asked.

"It wouldn't usually affect getting pregnant," he responded.

"I cannot prove it, but all the research I've done leads me to believe I might have a luteal phase defect," I said.

"If you did IVF, it wouldn't matter, because we would supplement you with adequate progesterone," he responded.

"What tests will be required and when?" I asked.

"We would start with FSH, LH, anti-Mullerian hormone (AMH), estradiol, and an ultrasound to determine your follicle count," he explained.

"From what I understand, if we attempted an IUI with injectable medication, at my age of thirty-six, my chance of conception would be anywhere from 15 to 17 percent, correct? If we did IVF, it would be a lot higher, right?" I asked.

"You have done your research," he joked. "Yes, a 15 to 17 percent chance of success for an IUI would be about right. However, the more important aspect is that your chance of having multiples would be 25 percent," he explained. "Our general IVF success rate is 50 percent, and the excellent success rate is 70 percent."

"My husband travels out of town every week, Monday morning to Thursday night. What is he required to do?" I asked.

"He will need to do a semen analysis and DNA fragmentation assay," he said. "He can do this when you both come in for the one-day workup. He also would have to be physically present for the egg retrieval, should you decide to proceed with IVF."

"Do you have any thoughts regarding why I might have miscarried so late in the first trimester?" I asked.

"The most common reason for first trimester miscarriages is genetic," he responded.

"Would we do a fresh or a frozen embryo transfer if we decided on IVF?"

"That would depend on how you responded to the medication. If your estrogen level was too high, or if you elected to do CCS, we would do a frozen embryo transfer," he responded.

"Can you explain the difference between CCS and pre-implantation genetic diagnosis (PGD)?" I asked.

"PGD is a form of genetic testing that allows couples at risk for single gene disorders to have embryos tested before a pregnancy is established. It can be performed for any pre-existing, known, inherited, single gene disorder. CCS testing is performed on a few cells biopsied from a Day Five embryo called a blastocyst to determine chromosomal abnormality. Waiting for the CCS results offers some time for your body to return to a normal hormonal state after ovarian stimulation. Studies have shown that transferring embryos into a uterus that is in a more natural hormonal state enhances the likelihood of implantation and a healthier outcome. After CCS testing, only embryos that have the correct number of chromosomes are selected for transfer."

"Who is a candidate for CCS?" I asked.

"Women thirty-five and older, a history of repeated miscarriage, a previous pregnancy involving a chromosomal abnormality, and multiple failed IVF cycles," he said.

"What is the miscarriage rate, despite doing CCS?" I asked.

"Approximately 7 percent," he responded.

"What are the most important factors for IVF success?" I asked.

"Uterus structure and embryo quality," he said.

My questions had been thoroughly answered. I walked over to the lab across the hallway, and had my blood drawn for the tests. Next was the "one-day workup." I had done a lot of research on the work-up costs prior to the initial consultation and was not thrilled to find out about the approximate out-of-pocket cost of $4,500. However, I felt this testing allowed us to cover all our bases, and potentially discover an underlying problem that was preventing me from becoming pregnant. Most importantly, I relied on CCRM's high success rate, and assumed the tests must be a contributing factor.

Two days later, Patrick and I drove to CCRM. After we checked in, the staff presented us with an intense one-day work-up schedule.

We sat in the conference room for the orientation with six other couples, feeling confident we had made the right decision. A nurse summarized all the information contained in the thick, three-ring binder we received at check-in. She made a point of reiterating the "gender selection" policy, reminding everyone that CCRM does not gender select. In other words, patients are not told which of their embryos are girls or boys, and cannot select which one(s) to transfer. This decision is solely up to the doctor, and is usually based on the quality of the embryo(s).

Semen analysis + antibody testing + chromotin assay

This was obviously Patrick's part. We needed to see if there was anything going on with the male reproductive side of things. Based on analyses in the past, I was not concerned that anything negative would be revealed; however, this was a more extensive workup.

Business Office

This is where we learned the financial costs. I was already well-aware of the fact that my current health insurance company did not cover any infertility-related expenses, including testing. I also recalled how I had been discriminated against, and ultimately denied health insurance, by a particular company due to "infertility." I was careful not to involve the insurance company in anything infertility related, so we paid for everything out of pocket. Insurance would begin to cover costs if and when I became pregnant. The business office representative estimated we could expect to pay about $21,000 for the type of IVF procedure we planned to undergo. This cost would include the one-day workup, egg retrieval, and frozen embryo transfer. But if the transfer failed, an additional transfer would be around $6,000.

This conversation was challenging to accept. If the first frozen transfer failed, we were looking at a grand total of close to $27,000. It was frightening to think about, especially since we could end up walking away with nothing.

Baseline ultrasound + Doppler

During this part, an ultrasound technician looked at both of my ovaries and reported that I had thirteen antral follicles on the left ovary, and eleven on the right. She commented that I had a "PCO-appearing ovary." Although she didn't conclude that I had polycystic ovarian syndrome, her comment did confirm my suspicion about having polycystic ovaries, which could explain the longer menstrual cycles. She also measured blood flow to and from the uterus, and reported that mine was "excellent."

When she left the room, I turned to Patrick and said, "So far, so good. So why haven't we gotten pregnant?"

"Well, hopefully they'll help us figure that out. That's why we're here," he said.

Nurse – IVF consult

Our assigned nurse showed us a demonstration video discussing how to administer the IVF injectable medication and explained the different types of medication the clinic might prescribe. She went over the important information regarding our upcoming cycle, and answered our questions. She appeared to be very organized, and seemed to have a "straight to the point" kind of personality, which is exactly what I needed from her.

Lab work and genetic screening tests

As a part of the standard workup, my husband and I were both tested for "communicable diseases," consisting of HIV, HEP B, HEP C, and RPR (syphilis). We also discussed genetic testing with a nurse, and decided to get tested for the most common genetic disorders of our ethnicities, which were cystic fibrosis, spinal muscular atrophy, and fragile X mental retardation syndrome. We felt the cost of this testing was minimal in comparison to the overall cost of IVF, and the results could be crucial for future decision-making.

Break

We had a 45-minute break for lunch and debrief.

"It's a lot of money," I said. What if it doesn't work? I don't like gambling."

"If we were to bet on a successful outcome, I think the odds would be in our favor," Patrick said.

"I agree, but how are we going to pay for all of this?" I asked.

"I crunched the numbers. We can do it," he said. "We'll have to scale back on certain expenses, but it's possible."

"Okay. If you're sure," I said.

I considered us fortunate. Infertility is expensive, and more often than not, health insurance companies exclude coverage. Many people are not able to afford treatments and are forced to try alternative ways to achieve pregnancy. Some people take out second mortgages on their homes, max out credit cards with high interest rates, and take out loans against their cars. Those who achieve success will often view the results as priceless, but those who do not walk away with a baby are often left feeling devastated, with a hole in their bank account.

Hysteroscopy

The hysteroscopy was a technique for looking at the inside of my uterus to diagnose fibroid tumors, polyps, intrauterine adhesions, and other pathologies. Before the procedure began, a nurse took my temperature. Because my temperature typically runs on the low side, I was curious what it was. When she told me 99.8, I flinched, and said, "Wow, that's definitely higher than normal. I wonder if I'm coming down with something." She reassured me that the number was in the normal range.

The procedure took about five minutes. Dr. Surrey assured us the future embryo transfer should be a "breeze," and he did not see any indication of C-section scarring.

Regroup

I looked forward to this part of the intensive day the most. We would have a chance to sit down with Dr. Surrey and discuss the bloodwork results. He came strolling into the office with a grin and a friendly handshake, just as he had done two days prior. He reiterated that the hysteroscopy was normal, and then revealed the bloodwork results. Knowing that most of the numbers looked normal, I immediately focused on the one that didn't: the FSH.

estradiol – 27
FSH – 9.6
LH – 5.5
AMH – 2.6

"How is it possible that my FSH was 5.5 only seven months ago, and it has jumped up to 9.6?" I asked.

I understood very well from my research that the higher the FSH value, the lower the chance of conception. Dr. Surrey explained that as long as the number is below ten, the chance of retrieving a sufficient number of eggs is good.

"Yes, but it's JUST below ten," I said. "What could have

changed in seven months? Could it be the difference from one lab to another?"

"We assume the highest number that's ever come back is the most accurate number. However, I don't see a problem with retrieving a sufficient number of eggs," he reiterated.

There was a lot to cover, so I decided to let this one go.

Dr. Surrey discussed the importance of having a mammogram before beginning the cycle, as fertility stimulation drugs can increase chances of developing breast cancer. I was not yet forty years old, and I was unsure if my insurance plan would cover the cost of a mammogram. However, I recalled the CCRM celebrity patient, Giuliana Rancic's, decision to move forward with IVF, only to discover that she had an early stage of breast cancer. We decided I would have a mammogram.

"I'm unsure what to do about CCS testing," I said. "I am thirty-six, but have had only one miscarriage, and I haven't had any failed IVF cycles. I also haven't had a pregnancy with a chromosomal abnormality. I'm aware that testing costs close to $7,000, so I'm leaning toward not doing it and taking our chances."

By the end of the regroup, we confirmed our decision to move forward with an IVF cycle without CCS testing, and Dr. Surrey said his nurse would create a "calendar" to get us started. He joked that this was the quickest he'd ever seen any couple make a decision. I laughed and said, "We want to move on with our lives. We made the decision months ago that if the three IUI attempts did not work, we would move on to IVF. We're ready!"

Fertility Lab consent review

This was our last meeting of the day. The lab representative discussed a twelve-page consent form, ensuring we understood its contents. The wording was straightforward, but some of it required insight and decision-making. My husband and I never considered, "The Ownership of Cryopreserved Embryos and Pre-Embryos, and the Need for a Disposition Plan."

No one likes to consider the possibility of a separation/divorce, death, or incapacitation, let alone what to do with embryos should one of these occur. Our options were either to discard the embryos, donate them for research, or donate them to another couple. We also had to decide what we would do with any extra embryos we decided not to use. After everything we had been through, I felt strongly about being able to donate embryos to someone or a couple who was not able to create them. My husband did not agree with me, and pointed out that our biological child would be "out there somewhere," and he wasn't comfortable with that. Much to my husband's relief, we would not be permitted to donate our embryos, because the maximum maternal age for donation was thirty-five.

As I waited for the HSG appointment, my nurse called with blood work and semen analysis results. As usual, every test result was "normal." Once again, we fit into the "unexplained infertility" category. The normal results were a relief; however, we were no closer to an answer as to why we hadn't become pregnant on our own. We hoped things would change now that we were about to begin the IVF process.

Six days after the one-day workup, I went back to CCRM for the HSG. I had an HSG approximately three-and-a-half years prior, so I was familiar with the actual procedure. I knew the HSG provides x-ray images of the uterus and fallopian tubes. It also can reveal abnormalities in the uterus that might interfere with pregnancy, such as growths of various kinds and abnormalities in the shape or lining of the uterus.

The friendly technician guided me to the x-ray office and took my temperature and blood pressure. I again asked what my temperature was, and she said ninety-nine degrees. I was baffled about why it continued to be higher than normal, but thought maybe it was because temperatures tend to be higher in the afternoon. She then led me to a bathroom where she handed me a cup for a urine test. When asked what this was for, she explained that it was for a pregnancy test, and that it was a standard procedure. It would be dangerous to perform an HSG on someone who was pregnant. I laughed and said, "Well, that's definitely not going to be a problem."

As I sat in the office waiting for her to return, I wondered what could be taking so long. She poked her head in the door. "Are you able to provide another sample for me? This test is coming up positive."

"What?" I exclaimed. "I don't understand. That can't be possible."

"Well, let's do another so we can rule it out. Maybe this one is a false positive."

I provided another sample and waited for the results.

When the tech returned, she sat down opposite me and said, "Jen, we did three separate urine tests, and they all came up positive. Congratulations!" she exclaimed.

I didn't know what to say. I couldn't speak. I was completely confused, frightened, and even a little hopeful. She walked me over to the laboratory, where I would need to have my blood drawn for hCG to determine if I was indeed pregnant. While waiting for the results, I called Patrick.

"I don't know what's going on, but apparently three different urine tests say I'm pregnant," I said. "I don't believe it though, because remember not even two weeks ago I had a heavy period."

"Do you think there's really a possibility you could be pregnant though?" he asked.

"Anything's possible, but the likelihood is really low. I just don't get it. I guess that's why my temperature was higher than normal. We'll have to wait for the blood test results."

My nurse called me back to her office, and we discussed what had just occurred.

"Jen, we got your blood work results back, and your level is 256. Congratulations! We consider you to be pregnant if the level is at least fifty. Yours is five times that," she said.

"I understand this is what the blood work indicates, but I just don't think this is a viable pregnancy," I said through tears. I then began sobbing. "My last IUI was three weeks ago, and I got my period not even two weeks later. I remember what my initial hCG level was when we conceived Liam, and it was definitely a lot higher not even two weeks later," I pleaded. "Trust me, I want to believe this is true. I really, really do."

"We'll do a repeat blood draw two days from now to see what the level is, and go from there," she said.

On the drive home, I became hopeful. Maybe the IUI had worked, and we were actually pregnant! Just as quickly as that thought formed, I thought about the heavy period and what I considered a low hCG level. Although I concluded there was nothing I could do about it, I went home and Googled "hCG levels." There were many stories of levels that had started off low and resulted in viable pregnancies. When I was almost finished with my research the next day, my phone rang.

"Well congratulations!" I heard Dr. Surrey say. "That was easy!"

"Well, no. Not congratulations," I said. I then went into the reasons this was more than likely not a viable pregnancy.

"Let's just wait to get the results back from tomorrow's blood test, and we'll go from there," he said.

My suspicions turned out to be accurate. I was *not* pregnant. The second hCG test showed that the level had dropped. In all the research I had done, I couldn't figure out what had happened. The only conclusion I could come to was that the two eggs I created had been released, and fertilized, but neither had survived. There was a possibility I had not produced (or taken) enough progesterone to sustain the pregnancy. Although I didn't have any proof of either scenario, it was what I allowed myself to believe.

It was necessary to continue having my blood drawn to make sure the level continued to decrease. The question then became: Who would monitor this? Would it be CCRM, or the facility that had done the IUI? My CCRM nurse and I agreed that it made sense to alert my previous facility about what had happened, and have it monitor my progress.

The facility agreed to support me by following my blood work results. Because I had a few blood tests that indicated decreasing hCG levels, I wouldn't be due for another test for a week. In the meantime, Patrick and I decided to take a break and planned a trip to Steamboat Springs, Colorado with a friend and his son. The morning we were due to leave, I drove to the facility for another blood test. The nurse called me soon afterward and urgently stated, "The hCG level has *increased*. You have to come in today for an ultrasound."

"Increased? Are you kidding me?" I had done enough research by now to know what this could mean. I clearly understood that an increase might indicate what is called an "ectopic pregnancy," where a fertilized egg stays in the fallopian tube. In rare cases, the fertilized egg attaches to an ovary or another organ in the abdomen. Ectopic pregnancies can require emergency treatment.

"Patrick!" I screamed from upstairs. "The hCG level IN-CREASED!" I gripped my cell phone, raised it in the air, and threw it across the room. "I can't take any more of this! I just can't!"

I delayed the trip to Steamboat Springs for a few hours for the necessary ultrasound. The doctor was empathetic while she explained what she saw.

"I think I see what looks like a gestational sac in the uterus where it should be located, but I cannot determine for certain, since it's so small and so early on. There is a lot of blood, so it's hard to tell. I definitely don't see anything in either of your fallopian tubes, but again, it would be difficult to know since it's so small."

"Does that mean I can just take misoprostol to flush everything out?" I asked. I had again done enough research to understand that this medication is used in place of a D&C when the loss occurs at such an early time.

"Well, no. The problem is, I can't determine for certain that this is NOT an ectopic pregnancy. If it actually is, the misoprostol will not be effective," she explained.

"You're not saying I have to take methotrexate, are you?" Again, from my research, I understood that this medication is routinely given to cancer patients and can have serious side effects, but it is necessary to treat an ectopic pregnancy.

"Unfortunately, yes. I cannot ethically prescribe misoprostol, not knowing if this is an ectopic pregnancy or not. If it is an ectopic, it could be life-threatening for you."

"Okay, I understand," I said. "How is this going to work?"

"We need to do a complete blood count test and get the results back before we can administer the medication, because it can have detrimental effects if anything on the CBC is abnormal."

"I hate to say this, and I know my health is the most important thing right now, but we're supposed to leave for a long weekend this afternoon. I wasn't expecting this to happen. Is it possible to do this all today?" I pleaded.

"We probably can get the CBC results back within a few hours. You would then come back to the office, and we would administer the medication. After that, you would continue to get your blood drawn to ensure the hCG level decreases," she replied.

I wept on the drive back home. I couldn't believe we were experiencing yet another setback. The biggest questions were why did this happen, and could it happen again? Worse, I was fully aware of how long methotrexate remains in your system, and since it is so toxic, I understood that our IVF cycle would have to be postponed.

I called my CCRM nurse, who confirmed the delay. After running my situation by Dr. Surrey, she said it would be at least three months before we could even consider doing the egg retrieval. Although I understood and appreciated the necessity of this, I was heartbroken. Three additional months of infertility felt like a year. However, there was nothing I could do.

Patrick and I discussed the pros and cons of doing CCS testing.

"Now that I've had a miscarriage AND a loss that can't be explained, I'm wondering if it makes sense to do the CCS testing," I said.

"I was thinking the same thing," Patrick replied.

"It's $7,000, which is a ridiculous amount of money on top of everything we've already spent. That means the whole thing could cost $34,000, give or take. However, I don't think I'm strong enough to go through another miscarriage. If we tested them, we'd be guaranteed the embryo wouldn't have any chromosomal abnormalities, so the likelihood of a miscarriage would be significantly reduced."

"That's true, but remember Dr. Surrey said there still is a 7 percent miscarriage rate, even with chromosomally normal embryos," Patrick said. "That said, I think your mental health is worth the cost of testing."

"I agree. Let's tell them we're going to do it," I said.

Over the next few months, I continued to get my blood drawn to ensure my hCG level was decreasing, and that the medication was doing its job. As mentioned earlier, I had gone out to dinner and had a few drinks with a friend the day my period started, not knowing I was, in fact, miscarrying. I called this friend after finding out what had actually happened, and she responded, "Do you think that going out that night had anything to do with it?"

I was confused for a second, but quickly realized what she meant. "Do I think having a few glasses of wine that night caused me to miscarry?" I asked.

"Well, yeah," she said.

"No. I definitely don't think that was the cause. Do you know how many people don't know they're pregnant and drink not just once, but multiple times, and nothing happens to the baby? No, I don't think that was the case," I said. It was yet another insensitive comment I did not appreciate.

It was April 2013, and the first anniversary of our miscarriage was approaching. I knew I needed a distraction. I believed that if I chose to stay home, I would end up crying on the couch and feeling like a victim. A trip to the Gulf Coast of Florida with one of my best friends Melissa allowed me to grieve in a healthy way. Although I *did* cry on the couch, I cried with a supportive and loving friend who listened and held my hand. We spent the remainder of the weekend taking long walks near the ocean and eating delicious meals. Each year the miscarriage anniversary date arrives, I will have these cheerful memories to focus on.

The fishing season in Mammoth, California was also approaching, and my in-laws had asked us numerous times to join them at their rented condo. We still had not disclosed that we were proceeding with IVF, and that we would have to remain in town for bloodwork tests and medication administration. We made a few excuses for not joining them, but then made the decision to disclose. We told them about the failed IUI attempts and the plan to move forward with IVF. As always, they were supportive and encouraging.

"Are you going to tell Chris and Erin?" Sandy asked. She was referring to my brother and sister-in-law.

"No. We're only telling a select few people," I said.

"Well I know they would be supportive of you guys," Sandy said.

"I know they would, but this whole thing is embarrassing, and the fewer people who know, the better." I began crying. "I know how much you guys would love another grandchild, and I'm so sorry we haven't been able to give you one. My heart aches for the baby I'm not sure I'll ever meet. I feel ashamed that my body won't cooperate," I said.

"Jen, of course you know we would love another grandchild. However, what's most important is that you take care of yourself. We are here to support you, and I know Chris and Erin will as well, should you decide to tell them," Sandy said.

I felt emotionally unstable, so I began participating in CCRM support groups. As an added benefit of being a

CCRM patient, I was able to attend groups twice a month at their offices on the weekend, at no charge. Patients could choose from either the "general infertility" group or "third party reproduction," and all groups were led by psychological counselors on staff.

The group I attended on a regular basis was led by a counselor who disclosed her infertility history, which I believe allowed many in the group to feel she understood us. The participants were both men and women, single and married, experiencing primary and secondary infertility, and some who simply had concerns about their ability to conceive. Often, I was the only one who already had a child, and I struggled about disclosing this fact. My heart broke for those who had not had a successful pregnancy and delivery, and I became even more aware of how grateful I was to have Liam. When I would disclose my status, my voice would shake, and I would look down at the ground. I would follow it up with the fact that I had taken medication to conceive my son, and all the losses we had experienced since then. It might have appeared like I was defending myself, and I probably was. Although there are supposedly more people who have difficulty conceiving a second child, we are far outnumbered in support groups by those who do not have any children. However, I was open to attending a support group because of my professional background. I understood it was not healthy to isolate myself, and I knew the importance of connecting with others who were experiencing some of the same feelings and emotions.

These support groups gave me a place to vent, cry, and remember I was not the only one. They gave me permission to openly discuss my concerns without being judged. They allowed me to feel understood by a group of people who were in the trenches of infertility, and helped take some of the burden of listening to me off of Patrick and my friends. The group was truly a lifesaver. I am so grateful to CCRM for recognizing the need for the groups and providing them at no additional cost.

I soon received a text message from a forty-one-year-old friend that she had miscarried at approximately eight weeks. Despite being supplemented with progesterone, multiple home positive pregnancy tests, and very high hCG levels, the ultrasound indicated the pregnancy was not viable. My heart broke for her. After several more attempts, with each pregnancy getting shorter in length, she finally was forced to stop trying.

This is what concerns me about the media portraying the endless possibilities of becoming pregnant in your forties. Although it can and does happen, biology plays a major role for a lot of women. The fact remains that a female's ability to successfully reproduce is highest during her twenties, and steadily declines from age thirty and beyond. Celebrities have a right to their privacy, but many of us are certain these children were conceived via donor egg or embryo, and the media coverage doesn't paint an entirely accurate picture.

As Liam continued to get older, I thought about the spacing between children and why I felt this was important to consider. I had read that kids who are spaced *fewer* than three years apart will grow up as friends. They will enjoy similar activities at the same time, and will often share friends. They also will compete more with one another. They will go to college mere months or a few years from one another, creating a more difficult financial situation.

Kids who are spaced *more* than three years apart will not always enjoy the same activities, and the younger one will tend to emulate the older one. Their friends will be different, but they probably won't compete with one another. They will attend college years from one another, allowing parents more financial freedom.

I humbly realized I didn't have the luxury of deciding how far apart my kids would be spaced. This was something I thought I could control, but I was wrong.

At one of many children's birthday parties, Patrick and I met a mom from my son's school who had also been on the infertility roller coaster. While I was watching Liam play with the other kids, Patrick asked her if she had any other kids. I considered it to be an insensitive question, but she didn't seem fazed.

"Oh no. He was our miracle baby," she kindly responded. "We were lucky to have him."

During coffee, this mom described IVF attempts through the facility we had used before CCRM. She had experienced an early miscarriage, a few failed IVF attempts, a successful pregnancy and birth, and another failed IVF attempt when her son was twenty-one months old. She felt strongly that a local hypnotherapist, James Schwartz, contributed to her one successful birth, and she lent me his book *The Mind-Body Fertility Connection.* I read the entire book, became convinced his philosophy would work, and scheduled a series of appointments.

17

THE EGG FACTOR

"Every life has a rhythm to it. The important thing to remember is that creating an interchange between the coming and going, the rising and falling, the peaks and valleys, is what balance is all about. Your life may appear to be out of balance when in fact it could be that the rhythm of life is changing, and you are right where you are supposed to be."
                                      - John St. Augustine, *Living an Uncommon Life*

It was time to think about the upcoming egg retrieval, which had been postponed to the end of July 2013. I ordered my first dose of injectable medication to become familiar with what the medication looked like and how to administer it. I had twice injected Ovidrel to force ovulation, and had been terrified each time that I would do it wrong or it would be painful. Patrick was still traveling for work and wasn't around to inject me. I could have hired a nurse to come to my house, but with two injections a day at $75 per visit, I convinced myself I could do it. I watched how-to videos online and learned how to get the dosage right.

It may appear counterproductive, but the first step in the IVF cycle process was birth control pills. The purpose was to "quiet" the reproductive system to put the doctor in complete control of the hormonal process. I received a "calendar," listing what was required each day leading up to the retrieval procedure. It was overwhelming.

Date	Instruction	Injectable Medication	Additional Injectable
June 14	Begin birth control. Patrick begin doxycy-cline (2 pills a day for 10 days)		
July 9	Take last birth control pill (24 total)		
July 13	Ultrasound and blood draw for estrogen and progesterone levels		
July 14	Begin stimula-tion medication	1 vial Menopur in a.m.	150 IU Gonal-F + dexametha-sone at bed

Date	Instruction	Injectable Medication	Additional Injectable
July 15		1 vial Menopur in a.m.	150 IU Gonal-F + dexamethasone at bed
July 16		1 vial Menopur in a.m.	150 IU Gonal-F + dexamethasone at bed
July 17	Ultrasound and blood draw for estrogen and progesterone levels	1 vial Menopur in a.m.	150 IU Gonal-F + dexamethasone at bed
July 18		1 vial Menopur in a.m.	150 IU Gonal-F + dexamethasone at bed
July 19	Ultrasound and blood draw for estrogen and progesterone levels	1 vial Menopur in a.m.	150 IU Gonal-F + dexamethasone at bed
July 20		1 vial of Menopur and Cetrotide in a.m.	150 IU Gonal-F + dexamethasone at bed
July 21	Ultrasound and blood draw for estrogen and progesterone levels	1 vial of Menopur and Cetrotide in a.m.	150 IU Gonal-F + dexamethasone at bed

Date	Instruction	Injectable Medication	Additional Injectable
July 22		1 vial of Menopur and Cetrotide in a.m.	150 IU Gonal-F + dexamethasone at bed
July 23	Ultrasound and blood draw for estrogen and progesterone levels; genetic counseling appointment	1 vial of Menopur and Cetrotide in a.m.	
July 24	Ultrasound and blood draw for estrogen and progesterone levels	1 vial of Menopur and Cetrotide in a.m.	
July 25	Ultrasound and blood draw for estrogen and progesterone levels	1 vial of Menopur and Cetrotide in a.m.	10:00 p.m. – inject Pregnyl 11:00 p.m. – inject 1st Lupron
July 26		11:00 a.m. – inject 2nd Lupron	
July 27	EGG RETRIEVAL	Begin doxycycline	

Total number of blood draws and ultrasounds = 7
Total number of round trips to facility = 8
Total number of injections = 32
Total number of oral pills = 43

The facility performed a "suppression check" ultrasound to measure my lining and check my resting follicles after I took the last birth control pill. Baseline hormone levels of estrogen and progesterone were also checked. The ultrasound revealed that everything looked the way it should. I had approximately fourteen follicles on one ovary, and fourteen to fifteen on the other. This indicated polycystic ovaries, possibly a reason for my consistent delayed ovulation over the years.

I soon began the injectable medication. Despite having watched the instructional videos, I injected the Menopur incorrectly. I became stressed and concerned. My nurse reassured me that the Menopur mistake was "totally okay." I confirmed with her that I was not allowed to practice yoga while taking stimulation medication, and I wasn't to get my heart rate above 140 beats per minute. I asked if I could walk around the park, and she said yes.

I injected a different medication, Gonal-F (150 IU) at night, which was much easier to administer, and I did it correctly. I began feeling confident again. I had to inject the medication while Liam was eating dinner, and he asked, "What are you doing?"

"I'm going to give myself a shot," I explained.

"Like when I go to the doctor and get a shot?"

"That's right!" I said.

"Do you hurt yourself?" he asked.

"No. It doesn't hurt."

"Will you have to use a Band-Aid?" he asked.

"I don't think so," I said.

I was impressed with the emotional intelligence he displayed at only two-and-a-half years old. In that moment, I felt blessed not only to have him, but also that he was at an age where he will not remember this process, and was not able to ask very in-depth questions about what I was doing.

A follow-up ultrasound determined my response to the medication. Liam came with me to the appointment, and behaved well. I felt guilty in the waiting room with him, again thinking that it might emotionally trigger patients without children. However, the nurse reminded me, "People have no idea what you have been through before this." I agreed. First, the nurse drew blood for estrogen levels. Next, the sonographer determined I had seven follicles on each ovary of a good size. They were all growing at a similar rate.

"Ideally you don't want a lead follicle to take over," she explained. "Also, your lining is at a seven," she said. I knew that was a fairly good number, and I didn't expect to hear it this early in the stimulation process. However, I also knew the frozen embryo transfer would not happen until September, when my lining measurement would *really* matter. The nurse I spoke with after the ultrasound said my progress was "awesome," which I was relieved to hear.

It became increasingly difficult to avoid injecting medication in front of Liam. Because I didn't lock doors, he came and went as he pleased. One morning, he woke up earlier than usual. When I walked in his room, he asked, "Are you happy?" and when we walked to the bathroom, he said, "Mommy, I love you." It melted my heart and started the day off on a good note. He was watching a PBS television show while I did my morning injection; however, that night he asked, "Can I watch you do the shot?" I allowed him to watch, as I had no other alternative than to say no and lock the bathroom door.

When I returned for a third ultrasound, the sonographer said I had seventeen follicles, and they were continuing to grow as a group. My nurse called to say I did not have to come in for the ultrasound and blood work the next day because everything was flowing smoothly, including my estrogen level.

Liam asked to watch me inject Gonal-F.

"Does it hurt when you do that?" he asked.

"Nope," I responded, even though it did hurt. I didn't want him to be afraid for me.

I injected myself twice a day, for a total of twelve times and then began injecting three times a day.

To celebrate Patrick's birthday, and to take our minds off of the retrieval process, we all went to a Cirque du Soleil show. I did not realize that the show could be scary for a two-and-a- half-year-old. We had to convince Liam to stay for the second half, which was not easy.

My abdomen soon began to swell. I hoped this was an indication of a large number of follicles! The fourth ultrasound revealed I had a total of thirty-three follicles, eleven of which were 12 millimeters or larger (18 to 22 millimeters are desirable at time of retrieval), and twenty-two that were 11 millimeters or smaller. I was told that the doctor retrieves all possible follicles, even if they are on the small side. This is just in case they grew larger, and happened to fertilize. I again felt very grateful to have so many follicles to work with.

My estrogen level was 1,224 picograms/milliliter. I was happy to hear that, as many women get up into the five and ten thousands, which is a dangerous place to be because of the possibility of ovarian hyperstimulation syndrome, in which too many hormones can cause your ovaries to become swollen and painful. I had watched Giuliana Rancic endure this on her reality show, and knew how atrocious it was.

We regrouped with Dr. Surrey to discuss progress.

"Your lining looks really good, and I expect to retrieve about fifteen eggs. All the others will probably be too small," he said.

"I keep getting concerned about progesterone levels after the transfer, assuming that this might be a reason for the early miscarriages."

"Trust me, you will be supplemented with plenty of progesterone, so that shouldn't be a problem."

"When do you think the retrieval will happen?" I asked.

"We might have to push it to Friday instead of Thursday. You might need an extra day of stimulation medication. We'll find out tomorrow after blood work results come in," he explained.

When we left the office, I commented to Patrick, "I like Dr. Surrey. He is kind, professional, warm, and friendly, but also has a 'scientific' approach that gives me hope that he really knows what he is doing."

A few days later, we took Liam to school, and headed to CCRM for a long morning. First was the ultrasound, which resulted in a HUGE follicle count. The technician counted somewhere close to thirty-five follicles, and said the doctor would remove ALL of them, which I found hard to believe. She said it appeared nineteen of them would be good candidates.

We moved on to my IVF physical, where a nurse practitioner asked questions, took my blood pressure, temperature, etc. to ensure everything looked good for retrieval day. We then headed to the Comprehensive Chromosome Screening (CCS) class. We learned that in my age category (thirty-five to thirty-seven), 40 percent of the embryos tested are predicted to be "aneuploid," which means "abnormal." Much to my surprise and delight, we also learned that if we have two of the same highest-quality embryos, it is possible to request a preferred gender. The meeting leader explained that although two of the same quality is a possibility, it is uncommon.

We then met with a genetic counselor who discussed our family history. She described our family trees as "benign," which really meant there are no red flags, and we are at a very low risk for genetic diseases. That was a relief.

As we elected to do CCS testing on our embryos, it was necessary to discuss the specifics. We signed an agreement with the fertility lab stating that we understood the embryos could be damaged, that there is an accuracy rate of 95 percent, testing may not produce a result, and gender information is not provided. Also, a chromosomally *normal* embryo could be misdiagnosed as chromosomally abnormal and not transferred, lowering the chance of pregnancy. A chromosomally *abnormal* embryo could also be misdiagnosed as normal, be transferred, and result in a failed implantation, miscarriage, or an affected pregnancy. CCRM was understandably protecting itself from liability.

When we disclosed that my husband has a maternal cousin who has Down syndrome, the genetic counselor said approximately 95 percent of cases of Down syndrome are caused by a random event of mis-division of the egg or sperm around the time of fertilization. Relatives (other than the mothers of Down syndrome children) of these individuals are not thought to be at an increased risk. CCS testing screens for Down syndrome, so we were not concerned.

Patrick would be forty-six at the time of the retrieval. She mentioned that anyone forty-five years or older falls into the "advanced paternal age" category. However, there are no tests available at this time for advanced paternal age prenatal screening or diagnosis.

Nothing that the counselor said raised a red flag. We understood the CCS limitations, and our genetic history could be classified as "normal." We were hopeful and eager to start the retrieval process. However, before we left the session, we discussed one last detail. At the one-day workup orientation session, the meeting leader had clearly stated that CCRM does not allow patients to "gender select." She meant that the embryologists and doctors do not inform patients of embryo gender, and the final decision as to which embryo(s) to transfer is the doctor's decision. Although we understood and respected this, we thought it wouldn't hurt to mention that we did indeed have a gender preference in case two of the embryos were of similar quality.

"I know CCRM does not practice gender selection, but I thought I could mention that we do have a preference if two of the embryos are similar," I explained.

"I can certainly make note of it in my report, and pass the information along to Dr. Surrey," the counselor stated.

"Okay. Since we already have a boy, it would be nice to have a girl," I said. "I don't have any expectations, because I am fully aware of the policy. It would just be nice if it worked that way I guess."

I began feeling guilty about requesting a specific gender. After all we had been through, why couldn't I hope for the healthiest embryo, despite the gender? I dug a little deeper with Patrick.

"Do you think it's awful that we requested a girl?"

"No, I don't. Before we even started trying to have kids, we both said we'd like one of each," he replied.

"But isn't it like playing God? I just feel like you're so blessed to have a son who you can really identify with, and I would love to have the same with a daughter," I said. "More importantly, there has been such a negative mother-daughter pattern passed through the generations on my mom's side, and maybe I think I can fix that by having a daughter."

"Yes, but there are no guarantees as to what type of a relationship you would have with her," Patrick said.

"I know, but I'd just like to be given the chance. I'd love to play girlie things with her, and have conversations about boys and things. I never got to do that with my mom."

"You don't have to feel that guilty. Think about the reproductive facilities around the world that allow patients to gender select. It happens more than you'd think," Patrick said.

"I'm amazed that it's as common as it is. I wonder if those who can afford IVF will do it just to be guaranteed a boy or a girl," I said.

"We'll see. I don't think your line of thinking is too far off!"

Later that afternoon, a nurse called to say it would be necessary to complete one more day of stimulation medication, an ultrasound, and blood work. This indicated that the retrieval would be delayed. My estrogen level was 2,059 picograms/milliliter. From what I understood, a level of 3000 or more could lead to ovarian hyperstimulation, so I was satisfied. I was still learning to let go of control, step aside, and just let the experts do their work. If they were concerned about something, they would let me know.

I received another phone call to purchase more medication because the follicles were not large enough for triggering. I spent $572 on one day of extra medication, in addition to $120 for the previous day, and another $155 for the trigger shot. I was becoming exhausted with all of the extra costs, and I hoped again that it would result in a baby. I could feel the swelling of my ovaries, but it still was not uncomfortable.

The fifth ultrasound was promising. The technician said she thought I would do a trigger shot that night, meaning retrieval would be in two days. Getting to sleep was a little uncomfortable either because of all of the follicles, or possibly the two scoops of ice cream I ate!

In addition to the double dose injection of Lupron, Dr. Surrey prescribed an hCG injection called Pregnyl to mature the follicles even more. Unfortunately, Pregnyl is an intramuscular injection that is given in the upper outer quadrant of the buttocks! My husband and I watched a video on how to inject it properly. He bravely injected me, and it stung, but not as terribly as I had anticipated. I really worked myself up into a tizzy beforehand. An hour later, I gave myself the first of two Lupron injections. I slept very well! The following day I gave myself a final injection of Lupron.

18
HOPE

"As you gradually train your own thoughts into those of positive expectation, as you align with thoughts of worthiness and Well-Being, as you align your true power by seeking good-feeling thoughts — you will no longer offer resistance to your own abundance. And when your resistance stops, your abundance will come. A flood of good-feeling ideas and possibilities will flow to you."

- Esther & Jerry Hicks

We dropped Liam off early at our friend's house. He seemed comfortable playing with his buddy from school, and did not protest as we left. We headed to CCRM and arrived by our check-in time. I was called back to "pre-op" while Patrick remained in the waiting area. They prepped me with an IV, took vitals, and discussed what the procedure would be like. The nurse was friendly, as well as the anesthesia guy, and I was able to talk briefly with Dr. Surrey. Before being wheeled into the operating room, they gave me some sort of relaxation medication, along with something that started making me groggy. I remember them dimming the lights, and asking me to scoot down toward the end of the table, and that was it. The next thing I remembered was waking up in the recovery area about forty-five minutes later. My head was foggy, and my vision a bit blurred, but I felt relaxed. I had mild cramping, which turned into slightly moderate, then back to mild due to the help of Extra Strength Tylenol. They brought in Patrick, and we discussed his part of the experience. I was given ginger ale and crackers, and I rested for a bit. The embryologist came in to tell us that twenty-six eggs had been retrieved!! We were really excited to hear that number, because it gave us an exceptionally good chance of having at LEAST a few normal embryos.

The embryologist explained how they retrieve the most "quality" sperm, inject a single sperm into each egg, and hope fertilization will take place. He said we should expect a phone call the following morning, confirming how many had fertilized. He expected about twenty-three to fertilize. However, the ones that actually survive are greatly reduced by the time of the next phone call, because the embryos have five more days to grow. He said he expected ten or fewer to make it to the point where they would be frozen. One of the most important phone calls would be the one in a week, telling us how many embryos survived, and the quality of each.

A nurse took me to the basement parking garage in a wheelchair, and we were free to go. We picked up Liam and were told he had a fun day. We stopped off at the pharmacy to get Tylenol and a few Red Box movies. To avoid overstimulation, I ate a very salty package of ramen noodles, turkey meat, salt and vinegar potato chips, and drank a lot of vitamin water. I had mild cramps, but overall things were good. I felt blessed that everything had gone so smoothly, and that I was in capable hands at CCRM.

The following day the cramping began, and I had to take it easy the rest of the day. I was bloated and uncomfortable by bedtime. I was worried about ovarian hyperstimulation syndrome, but after Googling symptoms, I was certain I wasn't experiencing it. The embryologist called and told us, out of twenty-six eggs retrieved, twenty-two were mature and twenty fertilized normally. This is a very high number, and we were thrilled! We looked forward to the next call, letting us know how many made it to the blastocyst stage, and how they were graded. We would then know how many would be CCS tested.

The cramping continued, and I felt physically challenged watching Liam all day while Patrick was in California. I did a lot of sitting on the floor and playing with him, along with watching DVDs. It was uncomfortable to walk any faster than a slow pace, so walking around the house was all I felt like doing. After nap, we went to the mall. But walking with the stroller was difficult, and I had to take it slowly. I began to feel better but anticipated being sore in the coming days.

Recovering from the egg retrieval was harder than anticipated. I looked like I was four months pregnant, and the cramping lasted five days. I knew it would all be worth it in the end, but I could not help feeling sorry for myself, for us.

When the cramping became intense, I cried about our journey. It had been a rough road so far, and we were not even near the end. I grieved for having to endure what millions of other women do not. I grieved for this process testing my relationship with Patrick and the relationship I was establishing with Liam. I experienced continuous anxiety and depression throughout this journey, and I felt these important relationships were being affected. I grieved for all the money we had spent that could have put Liam through at least one year of college!

It was a curse, but a blessing at the same time. I was now able to see how fortunate I was to have been put through this "hell." I learned a great deal about myself and my perfectionist ways. I became more empathetic with myself and others who were experiencing difficulties. I became humble, braver, more confident, and more determined. Even though I didn't know the outcome, I did know I was stronger for it. And I was going to go on to do great things, whether that meant healthier parenting, doing great acts of charity, or having a thriving private practice. I did not know, but I was excited for the future!

We were notified we had eleven embryos to be CCS tested. Since we could test ten without further costs, we froze the eleventh. It is an additional $500 each to test any embryos beyond ten. All ten were of AA, BA, and BB quality, with AA being the highest quality level. We looked forward to the call from Dr. Surrey letting us know the final report: which ones were normal and which were abnormal. He would then make the decision about which one to transfer. We were happy with the outcome and eagerly awaited the next phone call, but we were "cautiously optimistic."

I spoke with my nurse to ask her about the process leading up to the frozen transfer. She indicated that the transfer might not be possible until the end of October 2013 because of how busy CCRM was. Liam would be three years old, and it would be one and a half years since the miscarriage. I did not appreciate hearing this news, as everyone I had spoken to along the way (including my doctor) indicated it would be anywhere from six to eight weeks after the egg retrieval, which would be the end of September at the latest. Over the months, I had realized my nurse tended to be conservative and always conveyed the worst-case scenario. I decided to wait to see what happened.

In the meantime, I waited to get my period so we could get things moving again. I was no longer bloated, and felt back to normal. When my period did arrive, I was instructed to begin taking birth control on cycle day three and continue.

I was driving back from grocery shopping when I heard my phone's voicemail signal. I had missed a call from Dr. Surrey, probably calling with the report. His message said he was leaving the office for the day, and to call him tomorrow. My heart started beating fast, and I frantically thought *you wouldn't call a patient at the end of the day to report bad news, would you?* My anxiety started creeping in as I thought about the possibility of not having any normal embryos. I tried to convince myself this was an irrational thought and it was nearly impossible at my age not to walk away with at least one normal embryo. I let it go, and thought it might be to our advantage to talk to Dr. Surrey when Patrick could be on the call as well.

I left a voicemail for Dr. Surrey, promptly at 8:00 a.m. the next day, asking for a return call after 11:00 a.m., when my husband was due to be back from the airport. I hoped his flight would not be delayed or cancelled. Liam and I took a long bike ride and planned to be back by 11:00 a.m. On the ride back home, I shoved my phone into my sports bra, set to the loudest ring tone, and on vibrate. I was NOT going to miss this call, even if I had to pull over on the side of the bike trail to take it. Unfortunately, we got delayed and didn't make it back until 11:20 a.m., but Dr. Surrey didn't call.

After we waited the entire day for a return phone call and left a second voicemail for him, Dr. Surrey called around 4:30 p.m.

"Out of the ten we tested, six were normal," he said. "Out of those six, you have two perfect embryos, and the other four are A- to B+ quality. Out of the two perfect ones, the day five is a higher quality than the day six." Dr. Surrey was referring to how many days it took the embryo to grow to the ideal blastocyst stage.

"Are the two perfect embryos different genders?" I asked.

"Yes, they are."

"I know you don't do gender selection, but if there's a very small difference between the two, we have a preference."

"Remind me about your preference."

"We would like a girl," I said.

"That shouldn't be a problem."

I couldn't believe it. I assumed, but was not entirely sure, that the day five embryo (higher quality) was a girl; otherwise, he would have reminded me the facility doesn't gender select. We were in an extremely good position at this point, but I remained aware of the fact that we still faced a long road.

I left a message for my nurse to call back about starting my frozen embryo transfer calendar. She suggested a transfer date of October 1. I was disappointed, because it was always my impression that the transfer would occur six to eight weeks post-retrieval. My nurse was able to speak with the lab and get me in at an earlier date of September 18, but she did not sound pleased with me. She said the six to eight weeks is from the time the chromosome test results come back. When I reread the paperwork, it did indeed mention that. She was also quick to mention that CCRM does seven transfers per day during the week, and the facility was entirely booked up for the month of September. I felt awful for becoming agitated and realized the emotional toll infertility had taken on me. However, she emailed me my calendar, and I began researching medications.

19
PREPARATION

"Embrace this moment, put one foot in front of the other, and handle what's in front of you. Because no matter where your mind may roam, your body always remains here and now. When in haste, rest in the present. Take a deep breath, and come back to here and now."
                                                          - Dan Millman

In the weeks and months leading up to the frozen embryo transfer, I started preparing for the best possible chance for success. I incorporated both Eastern and Western philosophies, firmly believing that both have an impact. At times, I felt as if I was overdoing it, but it had been well over a year since our miscarriage at twelve weeks, and I had a deep desire for the procedure to work, so I could emotionally, mentally, and physically move forward with my life.

I attended five in-person sessions with hypnotist James Schwartz after reading his book. I reasoned that James's five-session, mind-body hypnosis model might help me work with some of the old beliefs that I had been carrying that possibly were preventing me from becoming pregnant. Although I had never done any type of hypnosis before, I felt strongly about what he wrote in his book. Part of my homework after each session with James was to walk myself through a visualization exercise in which I would imagine a successful outcome. The visualization helped relax my mind, reduce my overall stress, and prepare my body for the upcoming procedure. I also felt it was a way of setting up a positive intention with the universe. I visualized for approximately twenty minutes daily as part of my morning meditation.

Deep breathing was part of my daily meditation. I attempted to empty all thoughts from my head and focus on breathing in and out for as many counts as possible. This would last approximately ten minutes, before I would begin the visualization.

I wrote a letter to my future baby, telling him or her of the growing excitement I felt about him or her coming into our lives. I read this letter out loud daily in the immediate weeks before and after the transfer.

Months before the transfer, I started writing in a gratitude journal. Each night before bed, I listed five things I was grateful for, mostly things that had happened that day. This helped me maintain a positive attitude when I was feeling anxious about all the medication, the actual procedure, and the outcome.

I took many walks around the park near our house. I had been used to working out at the gym at a moderately intense level. However, I reasoned that walking would allow me to appreciate the beauty of nature and slow down my thoughts.

I tried as often as possible to listen to uplifting music, both in and out of the house. I understood the positive effects that music has on the brain. Since I had always enjoyed listening to it, and seeing live shows, this was an easy thing to keep doing.

I continued attending church on a weekly basis, where I was inspired by the messages and like-minded members. Whenever I experienced a defeating thought regarding the upcoming transfer, I fell back on those messages. It did not work every single time, but it helped lessen the anxiety.

I also attended a support group within the church called Sacred Sisters, where one of the participants offered an opinion about a future pregnancy, stating, "I just know you're going to get pregnant, and I have a feeling it's a girl." I was overjoyed and shared that we hoped for a girl.

Through RESOLVE, I found people who had created infertility blogs. I chose which ones to follow, selecting those that were most similar to my situation. Reading personal thoughts and stories from those who "got it" was pacifying. Infertility felt isolating, and I realized how many of us experienced it. Although I did not create one myself, I realized how therapeutic blogging about your experience can be, coupled with the overwhelming amount of support you receive from those who subscribe to your blog.

I continued attending the CCRM-sponsored support groups twice a month and became a regular. As time went on, I became more confident telling the truth about already having a child. I often was the one who began the group introductions, because I was considered a veteran by the leader. I would start off by saying, "I have a son who was conceived with medication." I felt safe and supported, and did not feel that any of the members judged me. I occasionally met up with a few of the women outside the group, thus allowing for even more sharing and support. One of the women became pregnant on her first IVF attempt, which solidified my confidence in CCRM's success rate.

I continued with weekly acupuncture sessions, increasing to twice weekly leading up to the transfer. Almost every time, the practitioner told me my Chi (energy) was weak. I wondered if that was because my blood pressure had always been on the low side, or if the medication was causing it. Perhaps I was more anxious than I realized. Despite this, I continued to attend, believing it was beneficial for my body.

I also kept the lines of communication open with Patrick, who held me when I cried, as I listened to his words of wisdom. I was so grateful to be married to someone who fully supported me, and vice versa. It felt like we were in it together.

"I have been thinking a lot about how many embryos to transfer," I said. "I want this to work, and know we have a higher chance by transferring two."

"Yes, but remember that we could easily have twins if we do," he said. "I'm not comfortable with the high rate at which that happens."

"Yes, and I'm concerned about the physical toll of a multiple pregnancy, not to mention the possibility of miscarriage, prematurity, and stillbirth. Also, I know we budgeted for only two children total, and a third would be extra challenging," I said. "This journey has been so emotionally difficult, and I just want it to be over, but I agree that transferring two is risky."

"I think it's better to transfer one the first and second times, then consider transferring two the third time," he said.

"I agree. I can't endure more than three frozen transfer failures. My gut tells me if it doesn't work by the third time, it's not going to. I'll be grateful for the one child we do have and move forward. I admire those who are willing to go to the ends of the Earth to have a biological child, but I am not willing to, and it feels reassuring to have an 'end point,'" I explained.

"Then three total attempts is the plan," he agreed.

I had never been to a palm reader, but had always been curious about it. I felt this was the perfect time to have my palm read. My husband was skeptical, but was mostly concerned about my emotional well-being if I did not hear what I hoped. I went ahead with it anyway, and the outcome was interesting. The reader said five babies were in my "lifeline" and three were girls and two were boys. I obviously already had a boy, but I didn't know the gender of the baby I miscarried. I also was unsure whether or not to count the non-viable pregnancy from five months ago. It didn't matter. When I left the session, I was convinced we would have another baby, whether it was a boy or a girl. My husband smiled when I told him the outcome, neither discouraging nor encouraging me.

A friend from my church mentioned a "mystic" that she and her friends had been to. I was not entirely sure what mystics were, or what they did, but after some research, I decided to seek him out at an upcoming metaphysical fair. During our twenty minutes together, he told me about two past lifetimes I had experienced, and how those might be contributing to my inability to become pregnant naturally. He also mentioned that he saw a diamond in my abdomen, and this meant positive things to come. When asked if he knew the future gender of our child, he stated firmly that it was a girl.

I walked away from the session feeling even more hopeful that the transfer would be successful. I was pleased that he thought it would be a girl, but didn't want to get my hopes up. Dr. Surrey never confirmed the gender of any of the embryos, so I was still unsure which one would be transferred.

A few weeks before the transfer, I enrolled in twice weekly Tai Chi classes. I understood that Tai Chi could help with energy flow and my general psychological health. It was a form of meditation and allowed me to relax more fully.

Finally (as if I hadn't tried enough already), I created a list of reasons why I felt this procedure would be successful. My intention was to remind myself of all of the positives when my mind began straying to the negatives:

1. Previous ability to produce enough progesterone during pregnancy
2. Previous healthy pregnancy
3. Previous live birth
4. Healthy son (without CCS testing)
5. Six chromosomally normal frozen embryos
6. Perfect AA quality embryo to transfer

7. Additional perfect AA quality frozen embryo as back-up
8. Unexplained infertility diagnosis
9. Age 36
10. No caffeine or alcohol
11. Eating fruits and vegetables and nuts and good fats
12. Multi-vitamin, folic acid, and vitamin D
13. CCRM success stories – I personally know of six
14. High progesterone level
15. Estrogen level within normal limits
16. Triple pattern lining
17. The chosen embryo is already hatching

20
GO TIME

"You are able to live with uncertainty, even enjoy it. When you become comfortable with uncertainty, infinite possibilities open up in your life. It means fear is no longer a dominant factor in what you do and no longer prevents you from taking action to initiate change."

- Eckhart Tolle

I became more agitated leading up to the transfer. We started working with CCRM five and a half months earlier. I felt I was in a holding pattern and like it had been this way for a long time. I was getting impatient. I didn't know how many more pregnant women I could see every single day, especially when I was at the park, zoo, Children's Museum, Botanic Gardens, grocery shopping, and many other places. They almost always had a kid who was three or younger by their side. Some days it felt simply unfair and overwhelming, and other days it raised my hopes.

I attempted to live as normal a life as possible, so I took

Liam to the park. Of course, there were three pregnant women there. I felt discouraged and teary eyed. I actually cried at the park because it was just too much, and Liam kept asking, "What Mommy, what?" It was tough when Liam witnessed me getting sad about it.

I continued doing yoga, self-hypnosis at home, in-session hypnosis, deep breathing, healthy eating, walking, and acupuncture. I cut out caffeine and alcohol, and I had only very limited amounts of chocolate. I tried it all, hoping and praying it would end in a positive result for us. No matter what happened, I could say I tried my best.

On a number of occasions, Liam would say either, "I'm getting a baby," or "You're getting a baby." When I asked him if it was a little girl or a little boy, he said, "A little girl."

I knew that he was perceptive, but I had a hard time believing that he was *that* perceptive. How could a two-and-a-half-year-old understand what Patrick and I had talked about? We didn't talk about babies; we talked about embryos. We talked about chromosomes, and retrieval, and eggs, and transfer. I couldn't figure it out. When Patrick asked him if he knew why mommy was taking medication, he responded, "She's having a baby." I was blown away. When I asked him why I'm taking medication, he said, "Because you're sick." He appeared to understand that we were working toward a baby, but didn't know I was taking medication to achieve it.

I treated myself to a deep tissue massage, in an attempt to release any stress and anxiety. When I briefly discussed my situation with the masseuse, he said, "It's gonna happen for you." I wondered how he could be so sure of this without knowing much about me. Either he knew something I didn't, or it was something easy to say. Regardless, I put it in my subconscious, hoping he was right.

When I finished birth control, I called my nurse to ask about receiving the flu shot. She then surprised me with the news that all the CCRM doctors decided to supplement frozen embryo transfer cycles with progesterone in oil (PIO). Every other day, beginning five days before transfer, I would have to give myself a shot with a long needle, in the upper outer quadrant of my butt. This was in addition to the three times daily vaginal progesterone insertions. I asked if this resulted in higher pregnancy rates but was not given a clear answer.

I had previously asked about the possibility of doing PIO shots instead of vaginal inserts because they were less expensive. I was told patients start on inserts and do shots only if necessary. I had gotten used to the idea of not having to stick a needle back there, by myself, when Patrick would not be home.

My nurse also mentioned that my thyroid and antibody (Indirect Coombs) blood work soon would expire, and I would have to do them (and pay for them) again. I had previously asked her if any of the test results would expire, and she said they wouldn't. I hadn't appreciated her attitude and demeanor over the phone since the very beginning, but I tolerated her. When I asked her a question about my calendar, I felt as if she were belittling me. I got fed up with it, but it was so close to the end I decided not to voice my concerns.

I was soon told that my estradiol level was too low, and I would need to supplement with more estrogen. It seemed as if one negative thing after another was happening. However,

I had blood drawn for a second estrogen check, as well as an ultrasound. The sonographer said my lining looked "perfect." I asked her if any C-section scarring would be a barrier to implantation. She looked surprised and said, "NO!" She explained it to me in a way that I could finally understand. Apparently any scarring would be higher than where the embryo would be placed, and they would have found any scarring when I did my one-day workup. I added this to my "Reasons This Will Work" list!

The day before the transfer, I went for a walk in the park and reminisced about our "journey." I couldn't help getting teary eyed when I thought about how long a journey it had been. How much hope, excitement, loss, heartache, anxiety, depression, anger, disappointment, and more hope I experienced, and now here we were—a day before the big day. I had done a fairly good job of staying in a positive place, but here and there those self-defeating thoughts crept in. I was certain, though, that I had done everything in my power for a good outcome.

September 18, 2013 - Transfer Number 1

I walked around the entire park and listened to some soothing music along the way. I felt relaxed and ready to move forward. Someone from the lab called to confirm that we intended to transfer a single blast, day six, 5AA quality. I said yes, and he said something about having a very good chance at success. He said the most important factor is that the embryo is chromosomally normal. However, I did realize that he said a day six, and not a day five. I understood that to mean the female embryo would be transferred instead of the male, because I knew that a day five embryo was better quality than a day six.

We dropped off Liam at school, and arrived at CCRM. I got my blood drawn for estradiol and progesterone levels. We then headed up to the second floor waiting area, where I filled out some acupuncture information forms. Unfortunately, I had forgotten our check book, and the acupuncture group did not take credit cards, even though it charged $225 for its services. My husband went to the ATM to withdraw cash while I filled out paperwork and received my first round of acupuncture before the transfer. A nurse handed me a Valium, explaining that it would "relax your uterus." Valium also put me in a restful place so I could truly enjoy the acupuncture session. It lasted thirty minutes, but it felt shorter, possibly because of the anticipation of the transfer.

Dr. Surrey arrived with an embryologist and a nurse. He confirmed that we wanted to transfer only one embryo, and we said yes. Patrick was especially adamant! The embryologist had wheeled in a huge machine with something that looked like an incubator, containing the embryo. They had magnified the embryo on a monitor so we could take a picture of it. It had already started hatching, which we knew was a very good sign. Some embryos have a thicker outer shell, so they require "assisted hatching" on the day of transfer, which could have cost an extra $1,800 or so. Luckily it didn't fall into that category. Dr. Surrey also mentioned the "thawing" process went very smoothly.

They tilted me backwards a bit, the nurse pressed on my abdomen with the ultrasound device to guide where Dr.

Surrey would release the embryo, she inserted the tube that would carry the embryo to my uterus, and then it was released. The whole procedure took three minutes! I rested for fifteen minutes and had another thirty-minute acupuncture session. I rode in a wheelchair to the underground parking garage, where a nurse reminded me to return in nine days for a pregnancy blood test. I tilted the car seat back, and relaxed on the drive home. The orders were for strict bed rest, getting up for the bathroom or a snack only, and going up or down stairs only once a day, for the rest of the day and the next.

I grabbed a snack and headed upstairs for bed rest. I still felt a little sleepy from the Valium when I received a phone call from a nurse who said my estrogen and progesterone levels were adequate. I was so grateful they changed the progesterone protocol before my transfer so I didn't have to worry about the level! The rest of the day and night were spent watching TV and reading.

21
THE WAIT

"The only guarantee in life is change. When you are lost in the promises of some distant future, waiting for the magical day when you will finally be happy, all your energy is draining toward some future event, with little left over for enjoying the here and now."
— Annemarie Greenwood & Marissa Campbell,
LIFE: Living in Fulfillment Every Day

The next day, Patrick took Liam to school, and started tending to my bed rest needs: hot water with lemon, reading material, snacks for later, and breakfast. I started feeling nauseated while drinking the water, and assumed it was because I was hungry for breakfast. However, the nausea got worse after eating (and watching Beverly Hills 90210 reruns), and I thought I might throw up. It came in waves, though. I tried not to think about every little thing I felt in my body, but the thoughts continued to arise, *"Were those implantation cramps? Could I really be feeling nauseated this early on?"*

On day two, I gave myself the progesterone shot. My hand was shaking a little beforehand, but I knew it had to be done. I had to use my non-dominant left hand to inject, which meant I had to turn my head all the way around to the left to see what I was doing. I knew I had to learn how to do it before Patrick traveled for work, and thought I'd give myself a couple of practice tries to ensure I had it down.

I used the morning to relax a bit more, just in case my body needed it. Technically, bed rest was due to end when I woke up, but I relaxed as long as possible. Patrick took Liam to the zoo, so I read and watched TV.

I received a text from a friend saying she placed something on my porch. When I opened the door, there was a bouquet of flowers and a card with the same inspirational words my sister-in-law had read at our wedding!

> *May the sun bring you new energy by day,*
> *May the moon softly restore you by night,*
> *May the rain wash away your worries,*
> *May the breeze blow new strength into your being.*
> *May you walk gently through the world and know its beauty all the days of your life.*
> - Apache Blessing

She signed it "Sending you love, strength, and hope!"

I was touched at her supportive gesture, especially considering that she had experienced a failed frozen embryo transfer only eight months prior. What a kind heart she had that she could look beyond her own hurts and be so supportive toward me!

As excited as I was about the possibility of a success-ful transfer, and grateful for supportive friends, I allowed the worries and doubts to creep in:

"What if this didn't work?

Should I be feeling cramping sensations?

Are my breasts slightly sore?

My breasts are slightly sore because I'm pumping a lot of pro-gesterone into my body.

Maybe they're not actually sore. I don't know.

What if I'm pumping all these hormones into my body, and I'm not actually pregnant?

I'm convinced I'm pregnant. It HAD to have worked. I have everything working in my favor! The conditions were perfect, and I'm a textbook perfect case!

I'm feeling a little more sleepy than usual. I think that's one of the first pregnancy signs.

It feels like there's something going on in my abdomen.

I've been on such a long journey, and we've spent SO much money. It HAS to work this time.

I got nauseated the day after the transfer for NO apparent reason. That has to mean something, right?"

The "two-week wait" was pure torture. Day four, and I had another five days to go. It was excruciating not know-ing one way or the other. I was hopeful, but fearful at the same time. I did my best to fill my days with distractions. I kept myself busy to fend off the self-defeating thoughts, but I continued running the same script.

I had a new thought that becoming pregnant and having a second child would feel like winning the lottery, but my odds of success were WAY higher than winning the lottery.

To get positive news would be liberating and thrilling. We tried SO hard to get to this very point.

I finally received the call from a nurse who said my pregnancy test was positive, but my hCG level was a little lower than ideal. She added that my progesterone and estrogen levels looked great. The low hCG number scared me, but she said she had seen successful pregnancies at that level. Still, I was afraid mine would not be one of them, and when I hung up the phone, I broke down in tears.

Dr. Surrey called not long after and congratulated me. I was triggered by the memory of hearing that same word just over five months ago, when the pregnancy was false and there was nothing to congratulate.

"I've spent the last ten minutes on the phone crying to my girlfriend," I said.

"Let's not lose hope. I've seen a baby boy born with a starting hCG level of eight. Your level is forty-seven, only three points below what we like to see, so try to think positively. We'll have you come in for a repeat test, where we want the number to increase by 60 percent."

"I thought it only had to double," I said.

"No, that's old-school thought. We do, however, want to see the number above one hundred three days from now."

When the call ended, Patrick was relieved. He always liked hearing the information straight from the doctor, especially if it was positive. I was not relieved. I felt in my gut that this wasn't right. I started noticing that the bloating in my abdomen had decreased, and my breasts didn't feel as big or swollen. Some of it could have been subconscious, and some of it could have been due to not eating lunch because I was so anxious about the call. That night I went in and out of crying spells and didn't sleep well.

The older Liam got, the more he became aware of how those around him were feeling. When I cried, he seemed to get overly concerned, asking what was wrong, why I was crying, and if I was okay. He would say things like, "I'm gonna give Mommy a hug."

Here was a perfectly healthy boy who my husband and I lovingly created with minor assistance not even three years prior. Here we were after three losses in only a year and a half. I just didn't understand it. All the conditions were perfect. I had done so much work on myself. I understood (or so I thought) the possible reasons for the other miscarriages. Never in my ENTIRE life, had something been this challenging or humbling. I needed to have meaning, and I couldn't grasp the meaning of this. I was being tested, and tested, and tested, and it was getting exhausting. I didn't know how much more I could take.

We took Liam to see *Thomas the Tank Engine* the day after the phone call. I didn't feel up to going, but I decided to go and be there for Liam. In the past, I chose to isolate myself and indulge in a private pity party that only made me feel worse. That day, I chose to participate, and it felt like the best choice. It was a beautiful fall day, with sunny, blue, clear skies, and a slight chill in the air. The sun felt invigorating, and Liam had a wonderful time. I was grateful to have my son, and began realizing just *how* grateful as time went on.

After *Thomas* we went to a couple's house for dinner. They had a four-and-a-half-year-old, and an almost three-month-old. I wasn't sure how I would handle it, but they were friendly, welcoming, and genuine. Toward the end of dinner, the inevitable question came up: "Do you plan to have any more children?"

"We'd like to, yeah. It's just not happening. It's been tough."

The wife disclosed that she miscarried before having their first child, and miscarried twice before successfully carrying their newborn. I was amazed by how many people endure this. It was all around me, and, as upsetting as it was, it helped me feel normal.

I reluctantly drove to CCRM for my second blood draw the following day. On the way, while waiting at a stoplight, I panicked. I felt short of breath, dizzy, and my heart raced. I took a moment to compose myself. When I got to the facility, I broke down as I got out of my car and could barely give the receptionist my name. When it was time to have my blood drawn, I cried some more.

After I returned home, we headed to church. Even though I felt down and out, attending church on a regular basis was important to me. I decided sticking with a regular schedule would help the time go by faster, and the service might even lift my spirits.

The message of the day was "What I Want My Grandchildren to Know," and started out with photos of the senior minister's grandchildren, one of which was a baby. I thought I might have to get up and walk outside. However, it turned out to be helpful. What I took away from it was "Pain passes," and "Get up and get back in the game."

Later that afternoon, I received a call from my nurse stating the hCG level had risen just eight points to fifty-five.

This was not a good sign. I scoured the Internet for stories about slow-rising hCG levels and ectopic pregnancies. It seemed once you had an ectopic, the chances increase for having another. I wasn't too positive about the future. She said to continue taking my medication. This was going to be a challenge for me, as I believed I was more than likely wasting my time and money.

While waiting to find out what was happening, I finished reading *The Gifts of Imperfection* by Brene Brown, which discusses vulnerability and perfectionism. This was the ultimate vulnerable position to be in. I could fight it, or embrace it, knowing things would move forward and everything would be okay again. I was in the thick of the pain, but chose to open my heart and be vulnerable instead of fearful.

I began to ponder why I desired a family of four so intently, and why it had been so challenging to accept a family of three. I grew up in a family of four, so this was a "normal" number to me. I also grew up with a brother, and wondered if Liam would be missing out if he didn't have a sibling. Four was an even number; three was an odd number. I also wondered how well my son would thrive if he constantly interacted with two adults and no children in our house. And finally, I thought about what society considers a normal-sized family, and the number I came up with was four. Although the number of families with one child is increasing, the majority remains two. I wondered if I was fearful of standing out and not feeling whole without two children.

A nurse eventually called with the third hCG result: nineteen. The embryo transfer had failed, but I was not experiencing an ectopic. I had a choice. I had a choice about how to react. I could wallow in the fear and pain, or get out of bed and choose to live life. I could choose to support and love Liam like he deserved. I could choose to react to others' pregnancy news with positivity and support. I could choose to remember that pain passes, and I will not be stuck in this place forever. I could choose to continue my spiritual practices instead of turning my back on them. I could choose to be patient and wait for answers and advice instead of Googling and coming to my own worst-case conclusions. I could choose to sit in the pain and be vulnerable.

I sent the following email to my family and closest friends who knew about the transfer.

> *Hello all,*
>
> *Please forgive me for sending a mass email. I simply don't have the energy or strength to contact you each individually with this update.*
>
> *It is with a very heavy heart that I tell you our IVF transfer procedure was not successful. We received the news last Friday that the pregnancy test was positive, but the hCG (pregnancy hormone) was below the minimum of what they'd like to see. The level eventually decreased, meaning it was a "chemical pregnancy."*
>
> *I have been simply devastated by this news. I am distraught that our dreams of having a family of four are moving further and further from reality. This is absolutely the most difficult ongoing situation I've ever faced in my life, and it has taken all the strength I have left to continue moving forward. Suffice it to say, I have never*

*been more grateful to have been blessed with
Liam. I am baffled how he even came into our
lives, and truly consider his birth a miracle.*

*Thank you all for the support you've given
along the way. At this point, we're going to take
the necessary time to grieve, and are not sure
what our plans will be moving forward. We will
more than likely keep them to ourselves this time.
Thanks for understanding.*

Love and light,

Jen

As I was about to hit send, I wished I hadn't told so many people about the transfer. But I got such an influx of encouraging words, I realized I had made a good choice. I was relieved that no one attempted to tell me the story of a sister, cousin, aunt, etc. who had gotten pregnant right before she decided to do IVF or adopt a child. Instead, they simply acknowledged my pain and indicated they were there for me. A few emails stood out as examples of the best kind of support.

One of my best friends responded, "Oh honey, I am so very sorry. I am here for you with whatever you need. I am not sure how to help, but just know you can let me know what you need and I will be there."

A therapist friend said, "I am so sorry. I can hear the tremendous pain in your email and have such a heavy heart for you. What courage it took for you to write that. I'm not going to give any platitudes, because right now there's not much anyone can say that is going to make you feel better. Just take the time you need to grieve this and know we're here for you whatever you decide to do next. I think it's even harder when everything looks so good in a cycle and it doesn't work. It's like WTF. (Sorry for the language, but sometimes that just sums it up best!) It's so hard to make sense of any of this. Of course, it doesn't make any sense, but it is our human nature to ask 'why'—and a part of the grieving process. Remember, there's a support group on Saturday if you think that would be helpful. And please let me know if there is anything I can do. I'm wishing you comfort right now. Please do what you need to do to take good care of yourself."

My aunt said, "Just want you to know you are both in our prayers always. Sending all our love your way today and always!"

Another best friend said, "I am so sorry. I can't imagine what you are going through, knowing how much this meant to you. I wish I had words of encouragement for you, but don't want to say something positive when I know you need to mourn first. I don't want to say all this in a text, so I will call you when I get home from work. Thinking of you."

A cousin responded, "Jen, I am so, so sorry for you and Patrick. I will be thinking about you, and know that if you ever want to talk, I'm an amazing listener. Hang in there. We are all here for you, whatever you need."

I went back to my old habit and researched reasons why the embryo failed to implant properly. I simply could not accept that three losses in a row were just "bad luck." But I didn't find any explanation I wanted to pursue.

To relieve some of my anxiety, I took a walk in the park. About halfway around, my thoughts overcame me, and I started crying. I was near the beautiful beds of summertime flowers on the west side of the park, so I went toward a bench to sit down. I felt the urge to be closer to the flowers, so I headed to the interior of the flower beds. I sat on the gravel, put my head between my knees, and sobbed. After a few minutes, I looked up at the flowers, and saw a butterfly. I thought my mind was playing tricks on me, so I kept staring. Sure enough, it was a butterfly. During this time, a song by the artist Adele came on my iPod. The lyrics were, "Whenever I'm alone, with you.... you make me feel like I am home again." I recalled the butterfly that had landed on my arm at the beginning of this year and thought this couldn't be a coincidence. Plus, in the eleven years I lived in Colorado, I had never seen a butterfly out in the wild. A sense of peace and tranquility washed over me, and I felt more positive and energized.

I then walked to a much-needed yoga class. I had taken a class by the instructor before, but she never started the class off with "sharing." The first person to share was a lady who said she had a four-month-old and a two-and-a-half-year-old at home, so she was just exhausted!

"Are you kidding me?" I thought. I was constantly being tested on my reactions, and her situation was the superb test. I was overwhelmed by the tests. Everyone who followed her said either that they were "fine" or that they "forgot to set their alarm clock" or that their "arm was aching a little bit."

Next, it was my turn. I could have lied. I could have made something up. But I didn't. I followed Brene Brown's advice by daring to be vulnerable and said, "I'm dealing with a loss this week, so I really need this class." During the class, the instructor tenderly touched my back while in child's pose. It was exactly what I needed, and instantly the tears started to pour. Time. Healing always takes time. Fearing the unknown was a task I fought on a daily basis, and it wasn't easy.

22
A BREAK

"Hope that is attached to a particular outcome is looking for pleasure but fishing for pain, because attachment itself is a source of pain. It is best to hope for an experience of life in all its fullness — a life that can embrace both joy and sorrow and still be at peace, because joy and sorrow are sure to come in this life."

                        - Marianne Williamson

When I got my period, my nurse said it wasn't considered a "real" period because of the chemical pregnancy. Our next frozen transfer was to be delayed so my body could "rid itself of everything." I set up a regroup appointment to discuss the recurrent pregnancy losses, share my ideas, and come up with a plan. I just wanted it all to be over. It was sucking the life force out of me.

I went to church to relieve some of the anxiety and frustration, and the minister discussed how debilitating worrying can be to mental and physical well-being. I realized how intensely I had worried about our situation, and how it had negatively affected me. He suggested the following ways to deal with worrying.

#1 RELEASE what we're holding on to. We are cutting ourselves off from our greatest energy flow when we worry. If we are holding "fear energy," the universe has to take this as instruction, and we will NOT like the harvest.

#2 – REPLACE with positive affirmations.

#3 – RESTORE to co-creator instead of victim. No matter what's going on, you can respond powerfully and trust the process. Worrying never changes the outcome of what you're worried about. It never feels better. Worrying is a habit of the mind.

I understood worrying was not supporting me, but I found it extremely difficult not to. I supposed this was one of the many reasons I was given this infertility challenge.

I took Liam with me to the regroup appointment with Dr. Surry. This time, I wasn't worried about what other people in the waiting room thought of me bringing my son.

"So far I've had a miscarriage at twelve weeks, a positive pregnancy blood test that turned into a loss, and now a chemical pregnancy. Should I be diagnosed as having recurrent pregnancy loss?" I asked.

"No. Technically you don't fit into the recurrent loss category, because there has been only one clinically diagnosed pregnancy. This means the last two were not detectable via ultrasound, so they are considered chemical pregnancies."

"Do you think I have an immunological issue?" I asked.

"I don't believe so. You already have been tested for antiphospholipid antibodies, and you don't have a family history of clotting disorder. I think the transfer was just a case of bad luck. Everything looked as it should before: lining, hormones, and a chromosomally normal embryo."

"What about an endometrial scratch, or therapeutic biopsy or scratch test, or whatever it's called for the next transfer?" I asked.

"We could certainly do one. It might increase the chance of implantation, because new white blood cells form in the lining after they are sloughed off," he said. "We also could check for underlying hormonal issues, such as thyroid antibodies and glucose intolerance."

"I just really thought we had a high chance this time, considering everything looked great," I said.

"I understand. However, a small number of my patients who transfer chromosomally normal embryos do not become pregnant. There is no explanation for this. Worst case scenario, it could be a fundamental problem with your uterus that I am not able to detect," he explained.

I had my final hCG blood draw, which should have been lower than five (the point at which someone is not considered pregnant). I felt confident when I left, believing if the thyroid and glucose tests were normal, and if we did the endometrial biopsy, we might just have a fighting chance. After all, we still had a "beautiful" day 5 (3AA) embryo to transfer, which was the more robust one.

I began taking a class at the church called "Beyond Limits" with one of my favorite reverends, Cynthia James. During a break, I nervously approached Cynthia, and when she hugged me, I broke down in tears.

"I just experienced a third pregnancy loss in a year and a half, and I can't control my emotions. I feel broken," I confessed. "I'm so scared that having a second child just isn't going to happen."

She sat me down, held my hands in hers, and explained, "I don't know if having a second child is what is supposed to happen for you. I would advise not focusing on having a child, but rather fulfilling your higher purpose." She then began an affirmative prayer treatment, focusing on the health of my womb, and praying on my higher purpose.

I needed to do everything I could to ground myself and my thoughts, and this class was the perfect place. I was even brave enough to stand up and announce my challenge to the class. Just as I was feeling proud of myself, a fellow student approached.

"I was just wondering, have you thought about adoption?"

I had dealt with similar comments in the past, so I was prepared for this one. "Yes. We have thought about that, but decided we are going to continue down the path we're currently on." I understood her question was innocent, but I yearned for the day when these types of questions wouldn't exist in my world.

I spoke with my nurse, who proposed a couple of different scenarios for when we would be able to embark on the next frozen embryo transfer. She said either mid-December 2013 or the end of January 2014. She said the endometrial biopsy would take place at the end of the cycle right before the transfer cycle. Patrick and I agreed that a mid-December transfer would be the better option. The sooner we could move forward, the better.

She also discussed the fact that our communicable disease testing results had expired, and we would be required to do them again, at a total cost of $760. This was challenging to accept, because I was 110 percent certain that in the last six months, neither my husband nor I had contracted any type of sexually transmitted disease. However, I realized and appreciated the reason for testing.

We came up with a plan: the endometrial scratch would be at the very end of October, and the transfer would be November 25, a few weeks earlier than I thought! My husband would be in town, and my in-laws would be visiting for Thanksgiving, so my mother-in-law could help take care of Liam and me during bed rest. It worked out perfectly! I appreciated my nurse's willingness to find a timeline that would work for me.

Liam turned three years old in the midst of our chaos. I considered him our "miracle son." I was baffled how he came into our lives, and grateful every day for his birth. I knew this struggle would be that much more intense if we didn't have him. We were blessed on that day, and every day. Patrick was traveling for work, so Liam and I celebrated by eating ice cream at our favorite local shop, Bonnie Brae Ice Cream.

The following morning, Liam's former school teacher took our yearly family photos in the park. Luckily, it was a great weather day, and she got some beautiful shots. Later that afternoon, we had a party for Liam's birthday. I felt blessed to have a third birthday to celebrate. However, it made me realize how time just kept ticking away, how my son kept getting older, how kids would be spaced farther apart, and how my husband and I kept getting older.

Patrick and I celebrated our five-year anniversary on October 11, 2013. The day we married, I was blissfully unaware of the challenging path we would walk. I had become humbly aware that life happens on its own terms, and was not something that could be controlled. I ensured our anniversary was a celebration of the love we shared for one another. We arranged for a babysitter, and headed to one of our favorite restaurants. It had been just over four months since I stopped drinking alcohol, but when the server brought us complimentary glasses of anniversary champagne, I happily indulged. I had also started a gluten-free diet, and fortunately the menu was agreeable.

Leading up to the transfer, Liam and I spent a lot of time playing at the park. The grandma of a little boy we had never met asked if Liam was my only child. When I responded yes, she said to her grandson, "Can you tell Liam what you're going to be this week?" When the boy didn't answer, the grandma said, "A big brother! My daughter is due in a few weeks, and I'm helping her out."

This triggered me on a few different levels. The first was the fact that the age spacing between the two children would be minimal. The second was the fact that I wasn't yet pregnant. The third was the fact that the grandma was so willing to step in and help her daughter in a time of need.

At the end of October, I had the endometrial scratch on my uterine lining to get rid of the "bad stuff." This would hopefully create a more receptive environment for the embryo to implant. I waited and waited for my period to arrive, and was told if my period didn't come in the next few days, the week of Thanksgiving transfer was not possible. It didn't arrive by cycle day thirty-nine. After a few long, back-and-forth discussions between my nurse and my husband, we decided to plan for a transfer after my December period.

After forty-two days, my period arrived. It was a relief, but also a disappointment. Even though I knew odds were slim that I'd get pregnant naturally, my mind sometimes convinced me there was a chance.

We decided on a January 2, 2014 transfer date, which meant we couldn't travel to California for the holidays. We hoped a new year would mean a new chapter.

Throughout this process, I had a lot of dreams. In one in particular, I wasn't sure if I was pregnant after the transfer. Someone near me had a Doppler, and offered to scan my belly. We heard a strong heartbeat: guh guh, guh guh. I asked her if it was a boy or girl, and she said a boy. I could also see that I was pregnant, due to the size of my abdomen. I didn't often analyze dreams, and it was emotionally difficult to do so then. The disappointment that came when I made an incorrect conclusion about being pregnant was heartbreaking.

I had another dream. This time I was holding an infant, and holding Liam's hand while we walked through double glass doors. I was smiling, and I was thinking how having two kids was enough. I questioned myself on wanting to have more. The dream felt so real. I wasn't sure if it meant anything. I hoped so, but I was cautious.

December 2013

I wanted to prepare as much as possible for the second transfer. I recalled having been introduced to the practice of

Reiki while living in New Zealand. Reiki is a Japanese technique for stress reduction and relaxation. It also promotes healing. I had my first Reiki/energy-clearing session with Reece at *Body Mind Energy Center*. I wasn't sure what to expect going into it, but I am glad I had it. We worked on past life and anger clearing, positive affirmations, and welcoming a future soul into my life. Afterward, Reece mentioned that she worked on clearing out negative energy that was in my liver, hips, and throat, and said my "third eye" was closed. She recommended another session before the transfer.

I began thinking about how much less concerned I was about my calendar this time. I assumed it was because I knew the drill. I knew the medications and how to administer them. Last time, I created my own calendar that I followed obsessively. I did not create a calendar this time, and I felt more relaxed. I recalled the conversation with Reverend Cynthia, and reminded myself to follow my higher purpose, not the desire for a baby. I read the book *The Best Year of Your Life* by the late Debbie Ford, and I followed her instructions to be broad about the life I wanted. I continued meditating for anywhere from thirty to forty-five minutes each morning before Liam woke up. I lost a lot of the fear surrounding whether a pregnancy would happen or not, mainly because I knew there was a chance it wouldn't. Before the previous transfer, I was really fearful of it not working, but I thought it would because of everything I had put into place.

I decided to start on the "organize my office closet" project I had planned to tackle during the Christmas holiday. I came across the manila envelope with medical records from my pregnancy and subsequent miscarriage in early 2012. I saw ultrasound photos, mention of a 175 beats-per-minute heart rate, and a sticker from the hospital that confirmed the loss. I realized why I had placed it on the highest shelf in my closet with materials I shouldn't need to reference. I hadn't thought about the folder in ages, and there it was. It brought me back to that dreadful day we found out at thirteen long weeks that our baby was no longer with us. I had forgotten a lot of the pain, or so I thought. A flood of tears came bursting out, but the sadness lasted for only a brief time. I picked myself up off the floor, and continued cleaning out the closet. Acknowledging the grief and moving forward seemed to be the answer. I would never forget, but I realized the pain had lessened.

Exercise was my go-to means to lift my spirits. At the gym one day, I was listening to music and watching the flat screen TV news. The headline, "Teenager gives birth to triplets and the father is a fugitive," popped up. It was one of those, *"You've really got to be kidding me,"* moments. I reminded myself to stop reading into those situations—the ones I can't make sense of. I knew the only way to truly accept them was through non-judgment, and by letting them pass as soon as I heard them.

When it came time for the communicable diseases bloodwork, I felt humiliated that I was an infertility patient. I felt ashamed that I couldn't conceive "the normal way." Most of all, I felt angry that we had to prove we hadn't gone outside our marriage and contracted an STD, and that we had to pay close to $800 to prove it. I let myself cry while Patrick and I engaged in a few back-and-forth text messages:

JEN: We are absolutely required to get the communicable blood work done.

PATRICK: Merry Christmas to us.

JEN: I am so pissed, sad, and feeling like a victim!

PATRICK: Me too. Looking forward to closure with this chapter.

I often forgot how our situation affected my husband, but I was reminded all too well with his comment.

Instead of wallowing in my bad mood, I went to the CCRM support group, where I continued to realize there are so many of us hurting. One of the women had had two miscarriages and found out she had an "inversion" of one of her chromosomes. Another found out she's a Fragile X carrier. And another had had a miscarriage a year earlier and miscarried twins just three weeks prior. I was heartbroken for everyone in the group. I was grateful we had each other for comfort, empathy, and support.

Christmas Day was not the way I imagined it would be. Back in September, I envisioned I would be approximately fifteen weeks pregnant visiting family in California, proudly announcing the news to my brother and sister-in-law. I had a fantasy that we would ask our doctor to write the gender of our baby on a piece of paper that we would wrap up and open on Christmas or New Year's Day. Now I hoped we could do this for possibly St. Patrick's Day, which of course wouldn't be nearly as meaningful. It was yet another Christmas without being pregnant. I was reminded of this when an extended family member offered me wine at dinner. When I said no thanks, she smiled half-drunkenly and said, "No because of...?"

I soberly smiled and said, "No, unfortunately not."

The whole family went to CCRM for the communicable diseases blood work, my cycle blood work, and a lining check.

I was pleasantly surprised when the technician said my lining measured at 9.1, about the same as the previous transfer.

Later, my nurse called with my blood work results and reported all were within normal limits. In preparation for the upcoming January transfer, I had a second Reiki session with Reece. Afterward, she mentioned that this experience was very different from the last one. She said she didn't have as much "clearing" to do and worked solely on "restoring" my energy. I felt lighter and more positive throughout the rest of the day.

We then went to the bank to have the "frozen embryo transfer agreement" notarized. The notary asked if I could believe how fast this year had gone, and how it was almost January. I told him I couldn't wait for 2013 to be over, and once again thought to myself how this had been the most disappointing and challenging year of my life.

2014

Relieved that 2013 was over, I hoped we were on to bigger and better things. On New Year's Day I participated in a group "Gong Bath," where approximately fifty of us laid down on the floor for an hour while experiencing a variety of gong sounds. It was meant to clear any negative physical, emotional, and mental blocks. The leader had a choice of many stones and crystals to hold onto or put on our chakras. He recommended a stone specific for fertility, one that happened to be in the shape of a heart. I put it on my naval during the bath. This type of activity was not something I would have considered in the past, but I felt it couldn't hurt.

Interestingly, that night's mid-week church service focused on clearing the chakras, and was led by Reverend Cynthia.

January 2, 2014 – Transfer Number 2

I had a quick thirty-five minute session with my acupuncturist before Patrick and I headed to CCRM. After the usual pre-procedure testing and prep, Dr. Surrey entered with his team. He confirmed that, once again, the embryo had thawed perfectly. I was able to sit up a little bit to see the embryo on the screen.

"Dr. Surry, it looks like the embryo hasn't started to hatch like last time," I said.

"That's because this is a Day 5, 3AA embryo, so it hasn't grown to the hatching point yet," he explained.

"Will it be able to hatch?" I asked.

"Yes. There is a hole in the shell for it to hatch out of."

I decided to accept his explanation and not analyze it. Just like the last time, it took about five minutes to transfer the embryo to my uterus. I then remained lying down, slightly inverted, for an hour. A nurse pushed me in a wheelchair to our waiting car outside and reminded me to come back for a blood pregnancy test in nine days. On the way home, I reclined the car seat and relaxed, feeling sleepy from the Valium. I rested in bed, took a nap, and read a book.

23
REFLECTIONS

"Life unfolds moment to moment, and each moment arises as a result of the moment that was surrendered before it. Life is a surprise that always arises out of the unknown. You can either embrace the unknown and live it fully and joyously, or resist it and live in pain, fear, and struggle."
- Eliza Mada Dalian

During bed rest, I reflected on what I had learned throughout my infertility journey, mostly things I wish I had done or thought of differently.

I had relied heavily on information obtained from the Internet to determine what might or might not be happening. I obsessively Googled symptoms, diagnoses, and test results, hoping to teach myself what I felt the doctors were not capable of teaching me. Although I believe in the power of knowledge, there were certain times I wish I had taken a step back from the research. For example, when I learned that our first frozen embryo transfer resulted in a lower-than-normal hCG level, my Internet searches led me to many successful pregnancy stories of levels that had started out even lower than mine. This gave me hope, and hope is always a positive thing. But in the end, the result was the same. It was going to be the same if I had done the research or not.

Interacting with fellow RESOLVE members was comforting during a time when I felt emotionally out of control. The women and men were able to relate to what I was going through on a different level than many of my friends and family. However, I sometimes allowed myself to be swayed by their opinions regarding what line of treatment I should pursue, instead of relying on my own doctor.

I often compared my story to everyone else's. I would read a book about an actress who tried to get pregnant for a few years and was successful with IVF on the first try. I would balk at the story, thinking, *"This person hasn't been through anything. She didn't experience failures or miscarriages."* I would then go online and read someone's complaint about her first IUI not working after trying to get pregnant for six months. I would think to myself that she hadn't been through anything yet.

Then others began looking at me the same way, like my struggles were minor compared to theirs. When I created a post on secondary infertility on the RESOLVE site, someone who did not have any children was quick to point out that at least I had one. I realized that competing with and judging others to determine who has it the worst is not productive. How far are we willing to go? Is someone who hasn't yet found a life partner worse off than someone who has, but who is struggling to have a child? Is someone selfish who has two children, but desires a third? I learned that we all have our dreams, and when they aren't fulfilled, we have a right to grieve, no matter what the dream is.

I also diagnosed myself based on how I was feeling physically. I allowed myself to believe something was wrong with my pregnancy with Liam because I felt "twinges." I believed I was in the safe zone with the second pregnancy because I didn't have any bleeding and was heading into the second trimester. I had hope that I was pregnant after the frozen transfer because I felt nauseated. It didn't mean anything until it meant something. All the worrying did not change the outcome of what actually occurred. I have learned to wait as patiently as possible until a final answer is revealed.

I became anxious prior to a nurse or doctor calling with important results or instructions. I glanced at my phone every five minutes to see if I missed a call, creating even more anxiety. Had I practiced mindfulness meditation more during these times, I would have lived more in the present moment. I would have focused on keeping my thoughts on what I was doing, rather than letting them wander to what the caller might say. I learned the message will be what it is, whether I worry about it or not.

I created more angst and disappointment for myself by projecting due dates. Once I was made aware of an IUI procedure date, I would calculate to try to predict when my baby might be born. On more than one occasion, I was excited to learn that a due date would be close to my or my husband's birthday, or the kids would be spaced a certain number of years apart, or I wouldn't be able to travel to an event because I'd be too pregnant. I learned to cease calculating to prevent the inevitable disappointment that resulted each time I got my period.

When I passed pregnant women, I would experience a wave of sadness, and sometimes envy, jealousy, and anger. Instead of being happy for them, and silently sending them blessings, I would wish it was my baby growing inside of me instead. It took some time to realize that their pregnancy status had no bearing on my ability to become pregnant. Over time, I worked up the courage to silently bless and wish them well as they passed by, allowing me to feel a sense of peace.

Invitations to baby showers were one of the most challenging aspects of my journey. On a few occasions, I turned down the invites, knowing I would not be able to handle the emotions it would bring up. I wish I'd had the strength to attend them and support those who I hoped would one day support me.

There were many times I was hard on myself for not being able to achieve a successful pregnancy. I allowed religious views, voices from the past, insensitive comments, and other programming to dictate how I felt. Over time, I learned to tune most of these out, and I have become less self-critical.

I spent the year 2013 fearful of making travel plans. I was required to be in town to pick up fertility medication, report to the office for an ultrasound or a procedure, prepare for a transfer, or get my blood drawn. This left little time to schedule long weekend trips or extended vacations. One of my biggest regrets is missing my cousin's wedding. We were close growing up, and I would have loved to be there and witness him take this milestone step. However, I had been so desperate to make the first transfer happen as soon as possible, I chose to do it in the first available time slot, a week and a half before his wedding. I couldn't travel, because I had to be in town for the pregnancy test. By the time we learned there was no pregnancy, it was too late to go.

I attempted to control outcomes by working hard to achieve results. I researched everything imaginable regarding infertility. I obsessively made certain I knew which medication to take when. I screamed, I cried, and I yelled about procedures not working. I worried about the future. I was finally able to grasp that no matter how hard I try, I just do not have control over what happens in my life. In ultimate defeat, I learned to embrace the unknown.

24
THE VERDICT

"Clouds come floating into my life, no longer to carry rain or usher storm, but to add color to my sunset sky."

- Rabindranath Tagore

I remained on bed rest for a few days. I read, I did crafty projects, and I watched a little TV. I got up only to go to the bathroom, to my office (ten feet away), and to the recliner chairs in front of the TV. A lot of people find bed rest boring, but I found it to be a great opportunity to just slow down. It was nice to have meals, snacks, and drinks brought to me. The only possible pregnancy symptoms I experienced off and on were mild cramps. I tried not to get too concerned about what I might or might not be feeling.

I recalled the day the butterfly landed on me in California at the Monarch Butterfly Grove was exactly one year ago. I wondered if this could mean anything, but reminded myself of all the times I thought this way in the past, and it ended up not meaning anything.

When bed rest was over, I went to the CCRM support group. There was a couple who had flown from Germany for treatment. I was again reminded how many people come to this facility from out of state and overseas, often as a last resort. They disclosed attempting nine fresh and frozen transfers over a three-year period. I could only imagine how much they invested emotionally, physically, and financially. I continue to be saddened by the lengths people go to have a child, and I hope the success rate increases with research and advanced technology. I also desire to see infertility costs decrease during my lifetime, as many of those experiencing infertility are unable to afford treatment.

During the two week wait, I met up with a friend for tea. I had not had caffeine in seven months, and was limited to the herbal tea menu. My friend had been battling a fertility challenge of her own. She was able to easily conceive her daughter when she was thirty-nine, but trying for a second resulted in two early miscarriages, and a chemical pregnancy—all within a year. I was grateful to have a friend who was empathetic to my situation, and vice versa. We had an amazing spiritual conversation that really brightened my day.

As for pregnancy symptoms, I felt as if this cycle was similar to the last. My breasts felt fuller, and I had mild cramping on and off. My goal was to keep myself focused on the present moment, knowing I did everything possible to allow this pregnancy to occur, and the rest was out of my hands.

While pulling into the grocery store parking lot, the song "Royals" by Lorde started playing. I got a sudden wave of nostalgia as I recalled living in New Zealand (where the artist is from) and being carefree. I began singing, realizing how much I had missed feeling like myself. I was laughing, smiling, singing, and remembering fun times at concerts, when all of a sudden I started crying. I then went back to laughing. The thought went through my head that this might all be related to pregnancy hormones. I then cautioned myself not to look too deeply into symptoms.

My mood soon turned sour. It could have been from dealing with a new health insurance debacle, but I also started feeling I might not be pregnant. I convinced myself I should be feeling more symptoms, and began thinking more about a back-up plan. I again reminded myself of the conversation with Reverend Cynthia. It was challenging. While hoping for my highest purpose was ideal, I felt I needed to know what to expect. I was caught off guard last time, causing unnecessary stress.

I chatted with my friend who experienced a total of five fresh and frozen transfers and had one child. When she asked how I was feeling, I said I had created back-up plans, and I just had to accept whatever happened.

"You're preparing," she said, meaning I was preparing myself for bad news, just in case. I wished I could look forward to results day with a positive attitude, but it was hard not to try to protect myself from the pain of disappointment.

January 11, 2014 - Test Day

I drove to CCRM for the hCG pregnancy test, and arrived early so I could make it to my yoga class later in the day. On the way there, the Beatles song, "Here Comes the Sun," came on the radio. I hoped this was a sign.

I went back to the lab for the test, and the nurse wished me luck. On the drive home, the first song I heard on the radio was, "Finally," by CeCe Peniston, which I hadn't heard since it was released in 1991. It's about finally finding a man, but I thought maybe, just MAYBE, it could be another sign because of the lyrics: "Finally it's happened to me, right in front of my face, and I just cannot hide it."

I used "acceptance" as my intention during yoga class. I was determined to accept whatever news came. After class, I looked at my phone and realized an "unknown/no caller ID" had tried to call twice. I knew it must be CCRM, but was shocked to hear from someone there so early. I didn't see any voicemail, so I tried to reason what the outcome might be. I was shaking the whole drive home. I mentioned the call to my husband and said, "We'll just have to wait for a call back."

Twenty minutes went by before I noticed there were two voicemails. I listened to the first, which said, "I was just giving you a call with your blood work results from today. Things are looking good, but if you want to go over the specific results, give us a call back. I'll try calling back again in a bit." I looked over at my husband and half whispered, half cried, "She said things are looking good!"

We listened to the next message on speaker phone which said "...I tried calling you earlier. I was hoping we'd get to talk in person, but that's okay since we can't. We got your hCG level back today. It looks great. It's at 194. The level at this point should be above at least 50, so that's a nice positive test. Your other hormone levels look good. So we'll re-check on Monday, and just continue with all your meds."

As soon as she had mentioned the hCG level, I jumped in the air and shouted, "YES!" My husband and I hugged and hugged. I was shaking, crying, and smiling. We both couldn't believe what we had heard. Liam asked Patrick what was wrong with me, and he said, "She's just happy!"

The first person I notified was Christina. When she became pregnant with CCRM's assistance, she texted "PREGNANT" to me, and I had been waiting to do the same, so I did! I then called my friend who experienced the five fresh and frozen transfers, and who has been an incredible support throughout all of this. She sounded genuinely happy for me, but I wondered after the call ended if this news would sadden her a little. How could it not if you're human? I intended to discuss this with her.

The third was Lindsay, mentioned earlier, who had success on the first try with CCRM, but had a very high-risk pregnancy. She and her husband were waiting to use a gestational carrier the second time around. We also called my in-laws to tell them the news.

We decided to wait for the second hCG test to tell anyone else, knowing full well things can change. We also waited to calculate the due date. I held off figuring out a specific due date because I just couldn't handle setting up another date that meant something, and then passed me by.

The morning of the second hCG test, we went to church. I was wearing orange, not only to support the Broncos in the playoffs, but to support myself. Since I learned a lot about the chakras, I knew orange represented the sacral chakra, which is where fertility and conception reside. It was nice to see many others in orange as well. The quote on the church bulletin caught my eye: "Success is neither magical nor mysterious. Success is the natural consequence of consistently applying the basic fundamentals." – Jim Rohn

I was extremely grateful we had gotten this far and hoped for an adequate second bloodwork result.

I drove to CCRM for my second test. About three hours later, my nurse called congratulating me, saying my hCG had tripled! I asked if that could possibly mean the embryo had split into twins, and she said we won't know until the ultrasound, but the number was "normal." I was, of course, ecstatic about the results, and I still could hardly believe it was happening.

We were unsure if our future held a live birth. However, I began thinking about what actually caused this "success." What were the basic fundamentals that I consistently applied to create the natural consequence of success? I listed the things I had done to achieve success, broken into two groups: Western and Eastern philosophies.

Western
- Highest-quality embryo
- Reproductive facility with a very high live birth success rate
- Light cardio and strength training
- Daily liquid iron supplement

Eastern

- Two Reiki sessions
- Gluten-free diet
- Gong bath
- Daily meditation / visualization / self-hypnosis
- Affirmative prayer
- Acupuncture twice a week
- Church class
- Yoga

I wish I could say our success was due to one or a few of these things, but we will never know. We'll never know if IVF was the magic ingredient, or if the Eastern methods above could have helped achieve a natural pregnancy.

I recalled that January day, almost a year prior, when the majestic yellow and black butterfly landed on my arm at the Butterfly Grove in California. I felt impelled to research the meaning of butterflies and was pleasantly surprised by what I found. Butterflies symbolize personal transformation and a life area in need of profound change or transformation. According to www.SpiritAnimal.info, the butterfly, "guides you to be sensitive to your personal cycles of expansion and growth, as well as the beauty of life's continuous unfolding. An important message carried by the spirit of the butterfly is about the ability to go through important changes with grace and lightness."

I also remembered the butterfly that appeared while I sat in front of the flowerbeds in the park, the week after we learned the first frozen transfer had failed. I now understood that this magical creature might have been relaying a message: to hang in there, keep on trying, and stay positive. The website goes on to state, "When the butterfly shows up in your life as a spirit animal or totem, it might indicate the need to look at a conflicting situation with more lightness and different perspective. This totem animal is symbolic of lightness of being and elevation from the heaviness of tensions."

I went to the pharmacy to pick up some extra estrogen patches, and was waiting in line when someone called out my name. It was Sara from the CCRM support group, picking up more medication for her upcoming egg retrieval. She asked if I was pregnant, and I told her the positive news. During our conversation, Dr. Surrey called to congratulate me. I expressed how I've found it difficult to be in the position of the one who's not pregnant yet, and I'm sorry if any of it affected her. I felt absolutely overjoyed with the news I had just received, and at the same time very guilty for having told her. I have since found out that her frozen transfer of two embryos resulted in triplets, because one of the embryos split. Although I was overjoyed for her, I was relieved I was not equally blessed!

When I got home, I took a home pregnancy test, just to take a photo of it! We had been waiting approximately 636 days for this moment. There was such a difference in taking the test knowing how it would turn out. I allowed myself to bask in the joy of being pregnant, and I let the news sink in.

25

CAUTIOUSLY OPTIMISTIC

*"The dark night of the soul comes just before revelation.
When everything is lost, and all seems darkness, then comes
the new life and all that is needed."*

- Friedrich Nietzsche

The months following the successful embryo transfer were filled with joy, as well as angst. I had ultrasounds at seven and nine weeks' gestation. Each time, I worried about losing another baby. I breathed a sigh of relief when I saw the reassuring heartbeat appear on the monitor both times.

I continued injecting progesterone, inserting progesterone suppositories, placing estrogen patches on my abdomen, taking oral estrogen, taking aspirin, and getting my blood drawn once a week to ensure adequate progesterone and estrogen levels. All medications ceased around thirteen weeks of pregnancy.

Gearing up for the thirteen-week ultrasound was the most nerve wracking. It brought back all the emotions I had experienced nearly two years prior. I had been cautiously optimistic since we got the positive news, and I braced myself for what we would see on the screen.

"Is there a heartbeat?" I asked right away.

When the technician said yes, and when we heard it, I loudly exhaled. I knew making it this far was great progress. We decided not to bring Liam to this appointment, because we didn't want to reveal the news to him until we were in a safer zone than last time. We also didn't want him to tell his teachers and friends at school, fearing we'd have to backtrack if anything happened.

Liam already was asking questions, saying things like, "Mommy, it looks like you have a baby in there. Do you have a baby in there?" and, "Mommy, why did you get this belly like this?" He was beginning to catch on, and we set a date to reveal the news to him.

We soon received the results from the first trimester blood screen, indicating all risk factors for genetic disorders were comfortably low. A genetic counselor from the CCRM embryology department called to confirm they had indeed transferred a male embryo, and we would be having a boy. When they asked what our plans might be for the four remaining embryos, I said there was a very small chance we would embark on another transfer, as the idea of adding a third boy to the family was not entirely appealing.

"I wouldn't be too quick to make that decision if I were you," she said.

"Why? Are you saying our next best embryo happens to be a girl?" I asked. "I know, I know. You can't tell me the genders," I laughed.

"I'm not saying anything, but I will say you wouldn't be disappointed with the outcome."

"Wait a minute. Are you saying all four of the embryos are girls?" I asked.

"Again, I'm not saying anything. However, I think you should really think about your decision," she said.

When I revealed the information I learned to Patrick, neither one of us could believe that out of the six normal embryos created eight months prior, five were girls. What are the odds? We would have a decision to make, but we knew we had a bit of time.

Soon afterward, Liam and I traveled to CCRM with hand-written cards and a bottle of wine each for my nurse and doctor. I also was sure to include a hand-written card for the laboratory, a place I felt was a large part of our success. It was oddly strange, but relaxing to be sitting in the waiting area with a viable pregnancy. Just over a year had passed since the first day I walked through the front door of the facility, and I was glad I would not be coming back any time soon.

About a week later, I received the following letter from Dr. Surrey:

"Thank you so much for your very kind note and gift. It has been a pleasure to work with you. I am delighted that all is going well so far. Please keep us posted on your progress. I hope that you have an easy and joyous pregnancy. Best wishes."

Despite having a normal pregnancy, I continued to experience anxiety regarding the health of the baby. We told only our very closest friends and family, deciding to wait until twenty weeks to officially announce it. I did order the same pregnancy journal I had thrown in the trash almost two years prior. Although I was anxious, I didn't want to miss documenting any of the important pregnancy moments.

I periodically visited the RESOLVE website to check on the progress of my "friends." I felt caught between two worlds: one where I was frightened about how my pregnancy would progress, and another where I had beaten infertility. I could have discussed my concerns on the "expecting" forum, but I felt guilty that I already had a child and was expecting a second. I instead turned to local friends and my husband for emotional support.

I wondered if I had made a mistake by deciding to work with a midwife again instead of a high-risk OB. Was I considered high risk because we had a miscarriage and two early losses? Was I being negligent by not being monitored more closely? When I approached it with my midwife, she explained there had been no red flags up to this point, but I was more than welcome to switch if needed. I reasoned that my challenge was getting pregnant and staying pregnant beyond thirteen weeks. Since we were past that, I dismissed all high-risk concerns.

When week sixteen arrived, I wondered when I would feel movement. I had felt movement with Liam right around this time, but it took a few more weeks until I felt it with this baby, due to having what's called an anterior placenta. We were vacationing in Puerto Rico around nineteen weeks when I began feeling more regular movement. This also was the time when we decided to reveal the news to Liam. I videotaped his reaction while eating dinner in a historic plaza of Old San Juan.

"It's April 19, 2014 today, and Liam is three-and-a-half years old," I said.

"Obama's in office," my husband joked.

"And we want to tell you something," I said.

"You know when you ask what's happened to mommy's belly? You know what's going on inside mommy's belly? Mommy's having a baby," Patrick said.

"Daddy? Can we put the baby's bed in my room?" Liam asked.

"Well, it has to be born first," Patrick replied.

"I'm gonna give my guitar blanket to her," Liam responded.

"You are? Well that's very nice, but it's not gonna be a girl. It's gonna be a boy. Mommy's gonna have a baby boy," Patrick said.

"What do you think?" I asked. "You're gonna have a brother!"

"Mommy, are we having a brother?" Liam asked.

"You're gonna have a brother in September," Patrick said.

"And I'm gonna be the brother?" Liam asked.

"Yeah. You're gonna have a brother, and he's gonna have a brother," I said.

"So what do you think about that? Are you excited?" Patrick asked.

Liam nodded his head yes.

"Mommy's gonna get bigger. Her belly's going to get even bigger," Patrick said.

"You were right when you asked if there was a baby in there," I laughed.

"And mommy? How about you get a circle necklace and you carry it?" Liam asked.

"A circle necklace?" I asked. "Well, what's really interesting is I was gonna get a circle necklace with both of your names eventually, and it IS in the shape of a circle. I'm not sure how you knew that," I said. "I like how you said you'll give him your guitar blanket. That's really nice! So you know which room is going to be his? The yellow one."

"But I want him in mine," Liam said.

"He'll sleep in our room for a bit. Then he'll go into the yellow room," I said.

"But I want the baby in my room," Liam protested.

"We'll have to see about that," I laughed. "Looks like our appetizers are here!"

The twenty-week ultrasound was less anxiety-provoking than the thirteen-week one, but I still was concerned. We told Liam he would be able to see his baby brother on a TV and would hear his heartbeat! I hoped beyond hope everything would check out okay. I couldn't imagine having to explain devastating news to him. Not when we'd gotten this far.

When the sonographer flipped on the screen this time, I didn't ask if there was a heartbeat. I could clearly see it on the monitor, and we could hear it too. The sonographer asked Liam if it sounded like a galloping horse, and he smiled and agreed. We waited patiently while she assured us the baby was growing normally. When we walked out with a DVD of the scan, as well as the black-and-white photos, Patrick turned to me and said, "What a relief!"

I agreed, realizing my anxiety level had just been taken down a few notches.

When we remodeled our house, we added an extra bedroom upstairs for a second child. It had remained a guest bedroom where I stored the clothes Liam had outgrown, as well as the toys he was too old to play with. There was no reason to frequent this room, but I purposely avoided it because it reminded me of what we didn't have.

I went in to organize the room and get it ready for our new baby boy. As I sat on the floor letting Liam's old baby clothes run through my fingers, I started to cry. There was a long period of time during which I wasn't sure I'd ever be sitting there, waiting to use those clothes. I wasn't sure I would watch another baby roll over, sit up, stand, and walk. As I sorted through the toys, memories of sitting on the floor playing with Liam came flooding back. I felt grateful I would be able to play with those same toys with another son. I felt grateful we had been given a second blessing.

Patrick and I had decided on both a girl's and a boy's name back when I was pregnant for the second time, before the miscarriage. We had easily agreed on Liam's name the first time, and we did the same for the second. Even though we knew we were having a boy, and hadn't changed our minds about the name, I still couldn't bring myself to call him by the name we had picked before. It was always "the baby" or "our boy." I was even unable to write his name in the journal I kept for him. Closer to thirty weeks, I became more comfortable saying his name when I talked to him, and was able to use it in the journal.

Despite my increased confidence, I found myself using humor to combat the underlying anxiety I was feeling. I attended a workshop at my church with author Neale Donald Walsch, the same author whose book was left on my table in New Zealand thirteen years prior. A participant sitting next to me mentioned my pregnancy, and I said the baby was moving around a lot while Neale was talking. She said, "Movement is a good thing!" I replied, "I know. He's still alive!" Those comments tended to slip out of my mouth possibly as a defense mechanism. I can only imagine what the lady must have thought, especially if she had never been through a loss. I realized in that moment that I will never again be blissfully unaware of what can go wrong in a pregnancy.

The month before the due date, I went out for a celebration dinner with my friend Katie, where she posed an interesting and important question. "Would you take it all back if you could?"

I thought about it for a moment before responding.

"No, I wouldn't. As emotionally and physically challenging as my experience was, I would not have become the person I am if every single thing hadn't happened. Because I had to wait to get pregnant, I was able to explore my underlying anger and forgiveness issues with my mom through therapy, books, and classes at the church. I wouldn't have had time if I was taking care of a baby. I would still be living with the pain. I would not be as empathetic to those who are struggling with their own challenges and losses. Also, I know for certain I would not have been a good parent to children who were only two years apart in age. I needed time to gain patience and explore my past. I am so relieved Liam will be out of the terrible two's and three's, that he is fully potty trained, and that he is sleeping through the night in a full bed. He will be so much more independent and will be able to help me with the baby. No, I wouldn't take any of it back."

Four weeks before our due date, a friend gave me the most meaningful "Blessingway" baby shower I could have imagined. A Blessingway is an old Navajo ceremony, which celebrates a woman's rite of passage into motherhood. Friends and family wrote wishes for our baby, and passed around images and quotes I could put up in the delivery room to support my intention for a successful vaginal birth after C-section. It was a different experience from the shower for Liam, which was more of a co-ed party to celebrate the baby. Not only did we celebrate the baby at the Blessingway, but we celebrated my journey for becoming a mother for the second time. Sandy and Pat flew in from California to help celebrate, and gave us a special gift: a baby blanket made by Sandy's grandmother that was once my husband's blanket. I was grateful that she once again supported me with such a meaningful and generous gesture. I imagined the day that I might do something similar for my daughter-in-law.

EPILOGUE

In the weeks leading up to the due date, I had a lot of practice embracing the unknown. To alleviate anxiety about what might happen, I kept an open mind by meditating daily, walking, and having acupuncture and Reiki sessions. My mantra became "the best possible outcome," and I refused to fixate on what might or might not occur. I stayed in the present moment as much as possible, put trust in my medical providers, and assured myself everything would work out okay.

In the early morning hours of September 17, 2014, I went into spontaneous labor. I spent a grueling twelve hours laboring to bring my baby boy into this world, and at 6:37 p.m., Graham Robert Noonan arrived vaginally. He was a whopping 8 pounds 0.5 ounce, and 20.5 inches long, and healthy. He was placed on my chest, and when our eyes met, I whispered "Oh my God, you're here. Oh my God. Oh my God." I cried tears of joy while Patrick embraced us. We entered the hospital a family of three and left a family of four. It was almost exactly one year to the day that our first frozen embryo transfer failed.

We flew to California for Christmas when Graham was three months old, and took a trip up the central coast to the Monarch Butterfly Grove. Two years prior, I stood in the same place, convinced I would become pregnant based on the butterfly landing on my arm. I learned life doesn't work that way. It doesn't give you concrete answers. It happens in its own time, on its own terms. It would have been delightful to know back then what I know now, but that would take away the mystery of life. As I held my infant son close to my heart, I reminded myself of the importance of embracing the unknown.

ACKNOWLEDGMENTS

Many people have been instrumental in the creation of *In Due Time:*

This book would not have been possible without the unwavering support of my husband, Patrick Noonan. Thank you for encouraging me, providing advice, and entertaining Liam so I had opportunities to write. Your faith in my vision allowed me to continue writing when I felt like giving up.

To Liam, our beautiful first-born son, thank you for hugging and kissing me when I needed encouragement.

Words cannot express my gratitude to all the ladies who shared their infertility stories with me. Your persistence, bravery, and vulnerability motivated me to put my story in writing, and allowed me to never feel alone.

Many thanks to Robin Colucci, my "get published" coach and neighbor, for teaching me the ropes and being the first to pick apart my manuscript. Your straightforward, no-nonsense approach was humbling, but necessary!

A big shout out to Polly Letofsky and her team at My

Word Publishing for navigating me through the perplexing publishing world!

To the beautiful and inspirational Reverend Cynthia James, I am forever grateful for your support and encouragement in recognizing and helping me reach toward the highest version of myself.

Lisa Bullis, acupuncturist at Pin and Tonic, thanks for providing affordable services and using your expertise to assist me in achieving pregnancy. And also a big thank you to Reece Leonetti, Reiki Master, at Body Mind Energy Center for not only healing my unsupportive energy, but also providing unconditional support and mini therapy sessions. "Bobby" is grateful as well!

To Wash Perk, my neighborhood coffee shop, an energetic thank you for providing outstanding beverages and food, as well as an ideal sanctuary for writing.

Dr. Eric Surrey, my reproductive endocrinologist at Colorado Center for Reproductive Medicine, thank you for helping me, and thousands of other patients, realize the dream of becoming a parent. Your gentle nature and laid back bedside manner, and your expertise in the reproductive medicine field, are an inspiration to many.

Thank you, Mary Wilterdink, RN, CNM, my midwife who acted not only as a professional caregiver, but also an inspirational coach throughout my vaginal birth attempt. I will forever hold your patience, encouragement, and kind words fondly in my heart.

And to Graham, my little miracle, I dreamed of meeting you for many years. I am so grateful to hear your infant grunts and cries as I finish writing this book. They are music to my ears.

BIBLIOGRAPHY

BOOKS

Brown, Brene. *The Gifts of Imperfection: Let Go of Who You Think You're Supposed to Be and Embrace Who You Are* (Center City: Hazelden, 2010).

Donald Walsch, Neale. *Conversations With God* (Book 1) (New Jersey: Putnam Adult, 1996).

Ford, Debbie. *The Best Year of Your Life* (New York: Harper Collins, 2005).

Krause Rosenthal, Amy. *The Belly Book: A Nine-Month Journal for You and Your Growing Belly* (New York: Potter Style, 2006).

Schwartz, James. *The Mind-Body Fertility Connection: The True Pathway to Conception* (Woodbury: Llewellyn, 2008).

Weschler, Toni. *Taking Charge of Your Fertility* (New York: HarperCollins, 2002).

WEBSITES

Colorado Center for Reproductive Medicine (CCRM)
     website, http://www.colocrm.com

Google website, http://google.com

Hypnobirthing website, http://www.hypnobirthing.com

WebMD website, http://www.webmd.com

RESOLVE website, http://www.resolve.org

Rocky Mountain Hypnotherapy website,
     http://rmhypnotherapy.com

Spirit Animal website, http://www.spiritanimal.info/butter-
     fly-spirit-animal

ABOUT THE AUTHOR

Jen Noonan is a Licensed Professional Counselor (LPC), born and raised in Chicago and holds a Master of Arts Degree in Counseling Psychology and Counselor Education at the University of Colorado Denver. She is an active member of the American Society for Reproductive Medicine, and volunteers her time to infertility organizations. She currently lives in Denver with her husband, Patrick, their two sons, and their cat Lois.

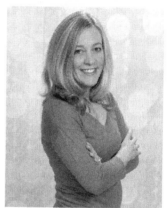

For speaking engagements, bulk buys, or simply to be a cheerleader, Jen can be reached through her website: www.induetimebook.com.

44696677R00150

Made in the USA
San Bernardino, CA
20 January 2017